# A Concise Introduction to

# MEDICAL TERMINOLOGY

*fourth edition*

*Carol A. Lillis*

**APPLETON & LANGE**
Stamford, Connecticut

Library of Congress Cataloging-in-Publication Data

Lillis, Carol., 1950—
     Appleton & Lange's introduction to medical terminology.—4th ed.
     Carol A. Lillis.

       p.       cm.
     Rev. ed. of: Brady's introduction to medical terminology. c1990.
     Includes bibliographical references and index.
     ISBN 0-8355-4321-9 (pbk. : alk. paper)
     1. Medicine—Terminology—Programmed instruction. I. Lillis,

Carol A., 1950- Brady's introduction to medical terminology.

II Title.

   [DNLM: 1. Nomenclature—programmed instruction. W15 L729a 1996]

R123.L7 1996

610'.14—dc20

DNLM/DLC                                 96–8407

for Library of Congress                     CIP

Executive Editor: Cheryl L. Mehalik
Production Services: Rainbow Graphics, Inc.
Designer: Libby Schmitz

10 9 8 7 6 5 4

Prentice Hall International (UK) Limited, *London*
Prentice Hall of Australia Pty., Limited, *Sydney*
Prentice Hall Canada, Inc., *Toronto*
Prentice Hall Hispanoamericana, S.A., *Mexico*
Prentice Hall of India Private Limited, *New Delhi*
Prentice Hall of Japan, Inc., *Tokyo*
Pearson Eduction Asia Pte. Ltd., *Singapore*
Editora Prentice Hall do Brasil Ltda., *Rio de Janeiro*

ISBN 0838543219

# Contents

# Preface

Why should you learn medical terminology? Many of you are continuing in health care careers and need this knowledge as a base for future study. Others, however, work or study in what may seem like fields unrelated to the medical world. An accountant, executive secretary, journalist, engineer, or even a lawyer may end up working for a company or institution in the rapidly expanding health care field. Almost any job may require knowledge of medical terminology at some time.

This text is geared toward the individual who has little or no previous exposure to the medical field. It is a basic *introduction* to medical terminology. It is not meant to be a complete anatomy text or a complete explanation of every medical condition! The text will, however, provide you with good word-building skills so that you can identify terms by their word parts. Included in this revision is an expanded unit, "Enlarging Your Medical Vocabulary." This unit covers medical financial terms that all of us need to know just to communicate about our personal health insurance coverage! It introduces diagnostic terms and tools, surgical terms and tools, along with pharmacology and oncology terms not in previous editions of this text. At the end of Unit IV are expanded lists of medical abbreviations and symbols.

You should take a few minutes to read "How to Use This Text" before continuing. The programmed format may be different from other texts you have used.

Individuals from all walks of life should find this text easy to understand and useful in their everyday lives as well as in their chosen career fields.

Thank you to Julia Guy, Linda K. Groah, and Miltex Surgical Instruments for the use of illustrations from their publications.

My deep appreciation goes to my family of Jim, Katie, Kyle, and Blair for their patience, help, and support during this revision. Contributions were also made by Dr. Louis Kartsonis, Scripps Memorial Hospital (La Jolla, California), and Diane Brown of Lee's Summit Physician's Group (Lee's Summit, Missouri).

*Carol A. Lillis*

# How to Use This Text

This is a programmed textbook that will allow you to participate in the learning experience by testing your knowledge on each bit of new material that is presented. If you master the material, you can continue. If you cannot grasp a section of information, you may be referred back to review before continuing to new material. The text works as follows:

1. You are presented with a single bit of information, which you need to master (a "frame" of material).
2. You are next questioned to determine whether or not you understand the information. Multiple choice questions accompany each frame with page numbers listed beside each of the answer choices. Select your answer choice, and turn to the page indicated. All answers are found at the end of each chapter in the "Answer" portion. You will also be asked to fill in blanks to test your recall and spelling skills.
3. If your answer choice was correct, the material on the "answer page" will verify this. However, if you selected an incorrect response, the answer page will provide additional information and either ask you to return to the page from which you came or direct you to specific remedial material.
4. You are not permitted to proceed to new information until you have mastered the preceding material. This method provides you with a more complete understanding of the subject matter once you have completed the text.

Occasionally you will be asked to fill in the blank with a term or definition. This practice encourages you to think about and spell the term correctly.

You will be given additional explanatory material whenever needed. Your rate of progress depends on your ability to respond correctly when questioned, and this ability directly relates to how well you learn the material presented in each frame. You are unlikely to complete the entire text at one sitting and may wish to take a chapter or part of a chapter at a time. The words repeated throughout the text are designed to reinforce your learning by using the same words to illustrate various elements of medical terms (ie, prefix, suffix, and stem). Exercises at the end of each unit test your knowledge before you move on. The answers to these exercises are found in the Appendix.

Word Element Lists are included at the beginning of each chapter and vocabulary lists conclude most chapters. At the beginning, only the word *elements* that are introduced in the chapter are included. At the end of the chapter, each complete word that was presented in the chapter is listed. These lists will assist you in reviewing the terms on your own.

To assist you in pronouncing the medical terms you will encounter in the program, a phonetic respelling of each term is shown in parentheses following the term. (The authoritative source utilized for determining the most commonly heard pronunciation is *Dorland's Illustrated Medical Dictionary, 28th edition.*) The phonetic respellings are presented in a simplified manner, using a minimum of diacritical markings (ie, markings used to distinguish or set apart elements of the term). A medical dictionary is a wise investment if you plan to remain in the health care field. Several are listed on page 278 (Additional Resources).

# Pretest

Before you turn to the first chapter, complete this pretest. Your pretest score will enable you to determine how much you already know about medical terminology. Record your score and compare it with the one you make on the posttest that you will take after completing the program. In this way, you can determine the effectiveness of your study effort. Write your answers on a separate piece of paper for ease in grading. The test answers are located beginning on page 256.

1. The three parts of a medical term are the prefix, stem, and _____.
   A. compound
   B. combining form
   C. suffix

2. In a medical term, the prefix comes _____.
   A. before the stem
   B. after the stem
   C. either of the above

3. The term **intravenous** means _____.
   A. around a vein
   B. within a vein
   C. beneath a vein

4. **Extracellular** means _____.
   A. within a cell
   B. beneath a cell
   C. outside a cell

5. The term **retrosternal** means _____.
   A. behind the breast bone
   B. to the left of the breast bone
   C. to the right of the breast bone

6. **Subcutaneous** means _____.
   A. adjacent to the skin
   B. beneath the skin
   C. within the skin

7. The medical term **pericardium** means _____.
   A. around the heart
   B. within the heart
   C. adjacent to the heart

8. Which of the following terms means **between the ribs?** _____.
   A. intracostal
   B. infracostal
   C. intercostal

9. **Before death** is expressed by which term? _____.
   A. postmortem
   B. premorbid
   C. ante mortem

10. **Preoperative** refers to which part of a surgical procedure? _____.
    A. the time period before the operation
    B. during the operation
    C. the recovery period after the operation

11. **Postmortem** means _____.
    A. before death
    B. after death
    C. causing death

12. The term **anesthesia** means _____.
    A. without sensation
    B. heightened sensitivity
    C. excruciating pain

13. A preparation used to counteract a **poison** is called an _____.
    A. antipyretic
    B. antialexic
    C. antidote

14. **Monomorphic** means having which form or shape? _____.
    A. a single form or shape
    B. many forms or shapes
    C. an unusual form or shape

15. The term **bicuspid** refers to a structure which has _____.
    A. a single point or cusp
    B. two points or cusps
    C. three or more points or cusps

16. In the term **triangle,** the prefix **tri-** indicates _____.
    **A.** one
    **B.** two
    **C.** three

17. How many letters are found in a word described as a **tetragram?** _____.
    **A.** two
    **B.** three
    **C.** four

18. **Multicellular** means composed of _____.
    **A.** one cell
    **B.** few cells
    **C.** many cells

19. A person suffering from a disease characterized by **polyuria** would void
    _____.
    **A.** urine tinged with blood
    **B.** a small amount of urine
    **C.** a large quantity of urine

20. **Hemiplegia** describes a condition in which there is _____.
    **A.** paralysis of one lateral half of the body
    **B.** paralysis of both sides of the body
    **C.** paralysis of the upper half of the body

21. **Hypertension** refers to _____.
    **A.** elevated blood pressure
    **B.** low blood pressure
    **C.** absence of blood pressure

22. **Hypotension** refers to _____.
    **A.** elevated blood pressure
    **B.** low blood pressure
    **C.** absence of blood pressure

23. The condition characterized by a **rapid heartbeat** is called _____.
    **A.** bradycardia
    **B.** arrhythmia
    **C.** tachycardia

24. In the term **bradycardia,** the prefix **brady-** means _____.
    **A.** sporadic
    **B.** slow
    **C.** rapid

25. Which of the following prefixes may be used to mean **white** in medical terms? _____.
    **A.** alb-
    **B.** alge-

26. **Leukocyte** refers to a _____ blood cell.

27. **Erythrocyte** refers to a _____ blood cell.

28. An **adductor** muscle is one which moves a part of the body _____ the midline.

29. The word **anteroposterior** would be translated as from _____ to back.

30. **Latero-** refers to the _____ of an object or body.

31. **Hydrocephalus** means _____ in the head.

32. **Dysuria** describes _____ urination.

33. **Dehydration** is a condition of the body where there has been an excessive _____ of water.

34. One or more letters or **syllables at the beginning of a word,** which explains or adds to the meaning of the rest of the term, is called a _____.

35. The **main body** or basic component **of a word** is called the _____.

36. **Lymphadenopathy** refers to a disease of the lymph _____.

37. **Dermatomyositis** describes an inflammation of the _____ and the muscles.

38. **Arthritis** refers to an inflammation of a _____.

39. **Myocarditis** describes a condition characterized by inflammation of the _____ muscle.

40. **Pneumonitis** refers to inflammation of the _____.

41. The term **myocardium** refers to the _____ muscle.

42. The term **gastroscope** describes an instrument used to look into the _____.

43. **Hepatitis** refers to an infection which is centered in the _____.

44. **Nephrolithiasis** indicates a condition commonly known as _____ stone or stones.

45. In a medical term, the stem **chole-** refers to _____.

46. The term **hematuria** refers to _____ in the urine.

47. **Lipoma** refers to a tumor which is composed of _____ tissue.

48. **Cholelithiasis** describes a disease state characterized by the presence of gall _____.

49. Used in a medical term, the stem **ren-** refers to the _____.

50. **Neuritis** describes inflammation of a _____.

51. **Osteoarthritis** refers to inflammation of a _____ and joint.

52. **Phlebitis** refers to inflammation of a _____.

53. A letter or **syllable placed at the end of a word** to add to its meaning is called a _____.

54. The term **hepatoma** describes a _____ of the liver.

55. **Lymphadenitis** refers to a condition characterized by inflammation or _____ of the lymph glands.

56. **Cerebrology** is the _____ of the brain.

57. **Hematemesis** describes a condition characterized by the _____ of blood.

58. **Inflammation of heart muscle** is described as _____.

59. **Inflammation of the lung** is described as _____.

60. **Polyuria** is a condition characterized by _____ urination.

61. **Leukopenia** is a blood disorder characterized by too _____ leukocytes.

62. **Dermatosclerosis** describes a condition which involves the hardening of the _____.

63. **Aphagia** is a condition which is characterized by the inability or loss of power to _____.

64. The term **appendectomy** describes the surgical _____ of the appendix.

65. The **excision of a portion of the colon** (or the whole colon) is called a _____.

66. Formation of an **artificial opening into the colon** is called a _____.

67. **Cystocele** describes a hernial _____ of the urinary bladder.

68. **Cystotomy** describes a surgical _____ into the bladder.

69. The **excision** of part of the intestine is known as an _____.

70. **Inflammation of the stomach** is known as _____.

71. **Hyperglycemia** refers to _____ sugar in the blood.

72. A medication to be given **a.c.** is given _____ a meal.

73. **Anemia** is characterized by a _____ of red blood cells.

74. A **muscle tumor** is called a _____.

75. **Nephritis** means inflammation of the _____.

76. A **hysterectomy** is the _____ of the uterus.

77. In surgery, the suffix _____ means to **form, build up, or repair.**

78. A **swelling in the tissue that contains fluid** is indicated by the suffix _____.

79. The position in which the **body and its parts are lying on their dorsal or back surfaces** is called _____.

80. The term used to refer to the **tail end of the body** is _____.

## MATCHING

Choose the word or words in Column B which describe the prefix, stem, or suffix listed in Column A. Some items in Column B may be used more than once.

**A**

81. Epi- _____
82. Endo- _____
83. Osteo- _____
84. Myo- _____
85. Arthro- _____
86. Phlebo- _____
87. Oto- _____
88. -emia _____
89. Mono- _____
90. Peri- _____
91. Nephro- _____
92. Hemo- _____
93. Hepato- _____
94. Arterio- _____
95. Reni- _____
96. Hypo- _____
97. Hyper- _____
98. Entero- _____
99. Encephalo- _____
100. Stoma- _____

**B**

a. eye
b. liver
c. intestine
d. wall of a structure
e. blood
f. ear
g. within, inside
h. kidney
i. muscle
j. bone
k. vein
l. joint
m. spinal cord
n. on, upon
o. below or low
p. artery
q. mouth
r. skin
s. midline
t. around
u. brain
v. posterior
w. above or high
x. one

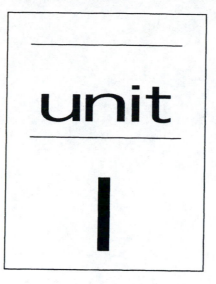

# PREFIXES

# Medical Prefixes

*Below you will find a list of prefixes to be introduced in this chapter. Similar lists will be provided at the beginnings of most chapters. They will preview material to be covered, and can also be used as self-tests. At the end of each chapter there will be exercises for review.*

## PREFIX STUDY LIST

| | | |
|---|---|---|
| ab- | ec-, ecto- | per- |
| a-, an- | endo- | peri- |
| ana-, an- | epi- | post- |
| ad- | ex- | pre- |
| ante- | extra- | pro- |
| ant(i)- | hyper- | re- |
| brady- | hypo- | retro- |
| co-, con- | inter- | sub- |
| contra- | intra- | super-, supra- |
| de- | mal- | syn-, sym- |
| dis- | para-, par- | tachy- |
| dys- | | |

The three parts of a medical term include the **prefix,** the **stem** or root word, and the **suffix.** You can tear down a medical term to find the meaning or create a new term by adding prefixes and suffixes to a stem. Not all words you encounter will have both a prefix and a suffix, but you can usually expect to find one or the other.

The word **prefix** is a good illustration of how medical terms are formed. **Pre-** comes from the Latin meaning before or in front of; **fix** comes from the Latin *figere*, meaning "to fasten." Therefore, the term prefix means "to fasten in front of or before." Prefixes are attached to the front of a stem to further the meaning. The prefix of the word **suffix** is **suf-,** which comes from the Latin *sub-* (also a medical prefix) meaning beneath, behind, or below. A suffix is fastened behind a stem to add to the meaning of a term.

Since prefixes and suffixes are attached to stems or root words, we will define these terms for you. Think of the stem as the "root" of the medical term. It is the base to which the prefixes, suffixes, or both will be attached to form a meaningful word. Every medical term will have a stem or be a whole word that can stand on its own.

# EXERCISE 1:

Prefixes are one or more syllables at the (1) _____ of a word or stem to explain or add to the meaning of the rest of the stem. The (2) _____ is the main body or basic component of the word and usually indicates the kind of tissue or body system which is involved. A (3) _____ is a letter or syllable placed at the end of a word to add to its meaning.

    a. (1) beginning, (2) stem, (3) suffix (page 27)
    b. (1) beginning, (2) prefix, (3) suffix (page 27)

There is no practical limit to the number of stems that may be compounded or combined to form a medical term, nor is the number of prefixes or suffixes that may be used with them limited. Take, for example, the following term:

**cardiopulmonary** (kar″de-o-pul′mo-ner-e)

This combines two stems to make one word: **cardio** (meaning heart) and **pulmonary** (meaning lungs)—pertaining to the heart and lungs. It has neither a prefix nor a suffix but still combines two stems to make a meaningful term.

Care must be taken to ensure that the meanings of the stems, prefixes, and suffixes are fully understood. The misinterpretation or omission of even a single letter may completely alter the meaning of a term—or even reverse it. For example, **hyperglycemia** (hi"per-gli-se'me-ah) (too much blood sugar) could be easily transposed to **hypoglycemia** (hi"po-gli-se'me-ah) (too little blood sugar) with perhaps disastrous consequences to the patient concerned.

Pronunciation of medical terms may also contribute to misunderstanding. For example, the terms **ilium** (il'e-um) (a bone-forming part of the pelvic girdle) and **ileum** (il'e-um) (the terminal portion of the small intestine) can easily be confused in oral use and even in written use where handwriting is involved. This is why it is important for you to learn the correct spelling and pronunciation of medical terms.

Let's begin our study of prefixes with the prefix **ab-,** which means away from or away. For example, the word **abnormal** (ab-nor'mal) is interpreted as:

| | | | | |
|---|---|---|---|---|
| **AB** | + | **NORMAL** | = | **ABNORMAL** |
| (away from) | | (state of balance) | | (away from a normal state; not in balance) |

Other medical terms incorporating this prefix include:

**ABDUCTION** (ab-duk'shun)—movement of a part away from the axis or midline of the body

**ABAXIAL** (ab-ak'se-al)—not situated in the axis of the body, away from the axis

The medical word **abductor** (ab-duk'tor) refers to a muscle that brings a part of the body away from the midline. In this word, as in abnormal, the prefix **ab-** means "away from."

# EXERCISE 2:

---

A medical term you may have occasion to use is **abortion** (ah-bor'shun). If we tell you the stem **or-** comes from a word meaning to be born, what would you say the word **abortion** means?

a. miscarriage (page 27)

b. normal birth (page 27)

The prefix **dis-** means apart, away from, or a separation from, usually in a negative sense. Look at these words:

   **DIS/ABILITY** (dis"ah-bil'ĭ-te)—not having the ability or being able to do
   (away from)                             something

   **DIS/INFECTION** (dis"in-fek'shun)—taking away any infection
   (separated from)


# EXERCISE 3:

Can you break down this word and define it?

**DIS/LOCATION** (dis"lo-ka'shun)—_____
_____

(See page 27 for answer)


The prefix **ad-** means to or toward, the opposite of **ab-**. Think of the word **adhere**—to cling together, to become fastened. Therefore, the words you just learned could read:

   **ADDUCTION** (ah-duk'shun)—movement *toward* the axis of the body
   **ADAXIAL** (ad-ak'se-al)—directed *toward* the axis


# EXERCISE 4:

An abductor was previously described as a muscle. What does the term **adductor** describe?

   a. a muscle that moves a part of the body away from the midline (page 27)
   b. a muscle that brings a part of the body to the midline (page 28)

# EXERCISE 5:

If we introduce the stem **ren-** to you, meaning kidneys, what would **adrenal** (ah-dre'nal) mean?

    **a.** near the kidneys (page 28)
    **b.** away from the kidney gland (page 28)

Another example:

    **AD/HESION** (ad-he'zhun)    to stick to; an abnormal joining of
    (to)  (to stick)            surfaces to each other

    Patients may sometimes suffer adhesions after surgery. In other words, certain body tissues or cells may abnormally be joined. The two surfaces would not normally be joined.

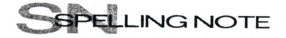

# SPELLING NOTE

Medical prefixes may vary in their spelling depending on the stem that follows them. For instance, the **d** in the prefix **ad-** becomes **s** if the stem begins with **s,** as in the term **assimilation:**

    **AS** + **SIMILATION** = **ASSIMILATION** (ah-sim"i-la'shun)
    (to)    (simulate or       (the changing of food into
           make like)         [or like] living tissue)

    The **d** in the prefix changes whenever the stem begins with c, f, g, p, s, or t. Don't try to memorize each exception to spelling rules just yet. It will be easier just to keep in mind that some prefixes *may* change their spelling depending on the stem, but it still means the same thing. If you find yourself having difficulty figuring out the meaning of the term because the prefix doesn't make sense to you, *then* you need to recall this information. A good medical dictionary will help. Sometimes you may find it easier to memorize the word, its spelling, and meaning as a whole, rather than breaking it down to prefix, stem, and suffix.

As you proceed through the text, we will explain other peculiarities of spelling medical terms.

The prefix **a-** means without or not, a negative prefix. Let's look at a few examples:

$$\begin{array}{cccc} \textbf{A} & + & \textbf{SEPSIS} & = & \textbf{ASEPSIS (a-sep'sis)} \\ \text{(not)} & & \text{(contaminated)} & & \text{(not contaminated or} \\ & & & & \text{clean surface)} \end{array}$$

It will appear as **an-** if the stem begins with a vowel or vowel sound in words such as:

$$\begin{array}{ccccc} \textbf{AN} & + & \textbf{ESTHES(IA)} & = & \textbf{ANESTHESIA (an"es-the'ze-ah)} \\ \text{(without)} & & \text{(sensation)} & & \text{(without sensation or pain)} \end{array}$$

Also meaning "not" is **in-**, as in:

$$\begin{array}{ccccc} \textbf{IN} & + & \textbf{SOMNIA} & = & \textbf{INSOMNIA} \\ \text{(not)} & & \text{(sleep)} & & \text{(not able to sleep)} \end{array}$$

$$\begin{array}{ccccc} \textbf{IN} & + & \textbf{TOLERANCE} & = & \textbf{INTOLERANCE} \\ \text{(not)} & & \text{(bear)} & & \text{(not able to withstand; sensitivity)} \end{array}$$

## EXERCISE 6:

The stem **phasi(a)** means speech. What would the word **aphasia** (ah-fa'ze-ah) mean?

a.  near the speech center of the brain (page 28)

b.  unable to speak (page 28)

# SPELLING EXERCISE

Decide which prefix (**a-** or **an-**) you would use to make the following stems negative.

1.  _____ pnea = not breathing
2.  _____ algesia = unable to feel pain
3.  _____ menorrhea = without menstruation
4.  _____ acidity = lack of normal acidity

(Answers on page 28)

The prefix **ana-** means excessive or upward. The second **a** is dropped when the prefix is used before a vowel.

An example of this prefix is **anaphylaxis** (an"ah-fĭ-lak'sis), an exaggerated allergic reaction of the body to a foreign protein or substance.

Another prefix which means above, beyond, extreme, or excessive is **hyper-**. You will see **hyper-** more often than you will **ana-** to mean excessive.

# EXERCISE 7:

Take the word **hyperactive.** What would you think it means?

a.  excessively active (page 28)

b.  hardly active (page 29)

Other examples of terms using the prefix **hyper-** are:

> **HYPERGLYCEMIA** (hi″per-gli-se′me-ah)—an excessive amount of sugar in the blood
>
> **HYPERTROPHY** (hi-per′tro-fe)—an overgrowth (excessive growth) or enlargement of an organ or part of the body (not caused by a tumor)

The prefix that means the opposite of hyper- is **hypo-**. The spelling can be critical to a patient's well-being if these two are misunderstood. **Hypo-** means beneath, below, deficient.

## EXERCISE 8:

From what you've previously learned, define the following terms:

1. hypoacidity (hi″po-ah-sid′ĭ-te) _____

   _____

2. hypoglycemia (hi″po-gli-se′me-ah) _____

   _____

(Answers on page 29)

## EXERCISE 9:

If we tell you the stem **derm** means skin, what would **hypodermic** (hi″po-der′mik) indicate?

a. on the surface of the skin (page 29)
b. beneath the skin (page 29)

## EXERCISE 10:

The stem **therm** refers to temperature or heat (think of a *therm*ometer). Which term would mean an abnormally low body temperature?

a. hypothermia (hi″po-ther′me-ah) (page 29)

b. hyperthermia (hi″per-ther′me-ah) (page 29)

Another prefix that means below is **sub-**. This is distinguished from **hypo-** in that it means beneath or under, usually in the physical sense. Take a look at the following examples:

**SUB/NASAL** (sub-na′zal)—below or beneath the nose

(below)  (nose)

**SUB/AURAL** (sub-aw′ral)—beneath the ear

(below)  (ear)

# EXERCISE 11:

Another medical term that means pertaining to the skin is **cutaneous**. Where would the **subcutaneous** (sub″ku-ta′ne-us) area be? _____

(Go to page 29 for correct answer)

Other frequently seen medical terms which use the prefix **sub-** include:

**SUB**  +  **LINGUAL**  =  **SUBLINGUAL** (sub-ling′gwal)

(under)      (tongue)          (under the tongue)

**SUB**  +  **AXILLARY**  =  **SUBAXILLARY** (sub-ak′si-ler″e)

(under)      (armpit)          (under the armpit)

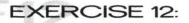

## EXERCISE 12:

Which of the following medical terms describes a disease condition that is somewhat acute, yet not severe enough to be classified as acute?

a. subarcuate (sub-ar′ku-āt) (page 29)
b. subacute (sub″ah-kūt) (page 30)

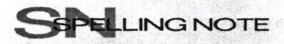

## SPELLING NOTE

The **b** in **sub-** will become an **f** or **p** if the stem that it is being used in front of also begins with an **f** or **p**. Examples are **suffix** (attached *behind* a word) and **suppedania** (an application to the sole [underneath part] of the foot).

The prefix that means the opposite of **sub-** is **super-** (or **supra-** in some cases). **Super-** means above or in excess of, and is similar to the prefix **hyper-**.

A "supersonic" jet goes in excess of the speed of sound (sonic).

**Superacute** (soo″per-ah-kūt) means extremely acute, very severe. Something that is **superlethal** (soo″per-le′thal) is more than enough to cause death.

More often, however, you will see the prefix **supra-** in medical terms. It means the same—above, beyond, superior.

## EXERCISE 13:

Using stems you have already learned, define the following words:

1. supranormal (soo″prah-nor′məl)_____

_____

2. supra-axillary (soo″prah-ak′sĭ-ler″e) _____

_____

(see page 30 for answers)

# EXERCISE 14:

Which of the following terms describes the surgical area of the abdomen that is just above the pubic arch?

   a. subpubic (sub-pu′bik) (page 30)
   b. suprapubic (soo″prah-pu′bik) (page 30)

While we are discussing up and down, another prefix needs to be learned. The prefix **de-** means down or from or down from in a negative sense. Look at a few examples of words that you should already know:

   **DE/COMPOSITION** (de″kom-po-zish′un)—the breaking down or separation of something (*not* putting together or composing an item or disease process, deterioration of a disease condition)

   **DE/CONGESTANT** (de″kon-jes′tant)—takes you away from being congested; it breaks down the congestion

   **DE/GERM**—disinfect (take away the germs)

# EXERCISE 15:

The stem **hydr(o)** refers to water. What would the condition of **dehydration** (de″hi-dra′shun) describe?

   a. submersion in water (page 30)
   b. removal of water (page 30)

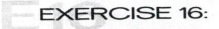

# EXERCISE 16:

Define the following terms:

1. deacidify (de″ah-sid′ĭ-fi) _____
2. decompression (de″kom-presh′un) _____
3. desensitize (de-sen′sĭ-tīz) _____
4. decontaminate (de′kən-tam′a-nat′) _____

(Answers on page 30)

Let's look at two more prefixes that have similar meanings: **anti-** and **contra-**. Both mean against or counter. **Anti-** means counteracting or effective against, whereas **contra-** means opposing.

Study these examples:

**ANTI/SEPTIC** (an″tĭ-sep′tik)—effective agent against sepsis or decay, germs

**ANTI/BIOTIC** (an″tĭ-bi-ot′ik)—counteracting life, specifically, the life of an unwanted microorganism

**ANTI/PYRETIC** (an′tĭ-pi-ret′ik)—fever-reducing; an agent that works *against* fever

**CONTRA/CEPTION** (kon′trah-sep′shun)—opposing conception

**CONTRA/LATERAL** (kon″trah-lat′er-al)—affecting the opposite side

# EXERCISE 17:

A word you will frequently see in relation to medications or treatments for patients is **contraindication** (kon″trah-in″dĭ-ka′shun). Which answer defines this term?

a. a condition or disease that would make the medication or treatment useless or harmful (page 30)
b. a medication given on opposite days of the week (page 31)

# SPELLING NOTE

The **i** in **anti-** is dropped before words beginning with a vowel, making the prefix **ant-**.

Although the word **con** in English means against, the prefix **con-** in medical terminology means with or together. There are words you should already recognize which use this prefix, such as:

CON/GENITAL (kon-jen′ĭ-tal)—born with

CON/CENTRATE (kon′sen-trāt)—to bring together to a common center or point

The prefix also appears as **co-** before vowels and the letter **h**, as in cooperate—to work together.

# EXERCISE 18:

You have already learned the word **adhesion** as meaning sticking together (abnormally). What do you think the word **cohesive** (ko-he′siv) means?

  a. working together (page 31)
  b. uniting together (page 31)

Other medical terms using the prefix **co-** or **con-** include:

CON/FLUENT (kon′floo-ent)—running together, becoming merged (together) (fluid, running)

**CON/STRICTION** (kon-strik'shun)—when something narrows together and
(together) (narrowing)                    is made smaller, as in constricted pupils
                                          or constricted blood vessels during a
                                          heart attack

## SN SPELLING NOTE

**Con-** becomes **col-** before words that begin with **l**, **com-** before **b, m** or **p** and **cor-** before **r.**

The prefix **syn-** (which also has a variety of spellings depending on the root word it's attached to) means with, along, together, and beside. A **syndrome** is a group of symptoms that occur together. There are many different types of syndromes, all with a special name that helps differentiate them from one another.

**Synovial** (sĭ-no've-al) fluid is a fluid that resembles an egg white and is found in certain sac areas of the body such as joint cavities, tendon sheaths (coverings), and bursae (tissue areas that otherwise would rub together).

**SYN + OVIAL =        SYNOVIAL**
(with)   (egg)     (with egg-like appearance)

## EXERCISE 19:

The stem **erg** refers to work. From what you've learned, what would you think the word **synergy** (sin'er-je) means?

a. working together (page 31)
b. looking like work (page 31)

# SSPELLING NOTE

**Syn-** appears as **sy-** if together with words that begin with **s**, then **n** changes to **l**, before roots of **l**, and to **m** before **b, m, p,** or **ph.**

Other words using this prefix are:

> **SYM/METRY** (sim′ĕ-tre)—a balanced arrangement of parts with reference to a center point; in good proportion
>
> **SYN/ARTHROSIS** (sin″ar-thro′sis)—a condition in which a joint is bound together; not movable

Some prefixes you will need to learn tell you about the speed of such things as your heartbeat or breathing. These are **brady-** (slow) and **tachy-** (fast, rapid). Some examples are:

> **BRADY** + **PNEA** = **BRADYPNEA** (brad″e-ne′-ah)
> (slow)    (breathing)    (abnormally slow breathing)
>
> **BRADY** + **CARDIA** = **BRADYCARDIA** (brad″e-kar′de-ah)
> (slow)    (heart)    (abnormally slow heartbeat)
>
> **TACHY** + **PNEA** = **TACHYPNEA** (tak″ip-ne′ah)
> (fast)    (breathing)    (excessively rapid breathing)
>
> **TACHY** + **CARDIA** = **TACHYCARDIA** (tak″e-kar′de-ah)
> (fast)    (heart)    (rapid heartbeat)

# EXERCISE 20:

Slow intestinal action would be described by the term (1) _____ -stalsis. Mental hyperactivity would be described by the term (2) _____ -phrenia.

a. (1)  tachy (-stalsis)      (2)  brady (-phrenia) (page 31)
b. (1)  brady (-stalsis)      (2)  tachy (-phrenia) (page 32)

Several prefixes indicate out, outside of, or out from. They include:

| PREFIX | MEANING | EXAMPLE | |
|---|---|---|---|
| e- | out from | **E/LIMINATION** (out from)   (threshold) | expulsion from the body (the threshold in this case) |
| ec- | out of | **EC/CENTRIC** (out of)    (center) | away from a center point |
| ecto- | outside | **ECTO/DERM** (ek′to-derm) (outside)    (skin) | the outermost layer of skin |
| ex(o)- | away from, outside, without, to remove | **EX/PECTOR/ATION** (out)    (chest) (ek-spek″to-ra′shun) | expulsion of mucus from the lungs |
| extra- | outside of, beyond, in addition | **EXTRA/CELLULAR** (outside of)    (cells) (eks″trah-sel′u-lar) | outside a cell |

## EXERCISE 21:

From the prefixes you just learned, see if you can define the following terms:

1. extracardial (eks″trah-kar′de-al) _____
2. exocrine (ek′so-krin) secretion _____
3. extracranial (eks″trah-kra′ne-al) _____ of the skull
4. extubate (eks-tu′bāt) _____ of a tube

(Answers on page 32)

# EXERCISE 22:

Which of the following terms describes a toxin (toxic substance) formed by bacteria that is found outside the bacterial cell?

a. exostosis (ek"sos-to'sis) (page 32)
b. exotoxin (ek"so-tok'sin) (page 32)
c. exoserosis (ek"so-se-ro'sis) (page 33)

How does one decide which is the correct prefix to use with a term? Again, it primarily means you must learn the words as a whole. This introduction allows you to be able to recognize any new term that uses these prefixes by already knowing what the prefix means.

The prefix that means the opposite of **exo-, ecto-,** etc. is **end(o)-. End(o)-** means within, inside, inner. Let's put **endo-** instead of **ex-** in front of the stems you just learned:

**ENDO/DERM** (also entoderm) (en'do-derm)—the innermost layer of skin
(inside)  (skin)                                in an embryo
**ENDO/CELLULAR** (en"do-sel'u-lar)—within a cell
  (inside)  (cell)

# EXERCISE 23:

You've already seen the term **exotoxin.** What would the term **endotoxin** (en"do-tok'sin) mean?

a. a toxin found inside the bacterial cell (page 33)
b. a toxin found on the outer edge of a bacterial cell (page 33)

# EXERCISE 24:

---

Where would an **endotracheal** (en"do-tra'ke-al) tube be placed? _____ the trachea (windpipe)

(Answer on page 33)

Another prefix which means within is **intra-,** as in the word **intramuscular** (in"trah-mus'ku-lar):

      **INTRA + MUSCULAR = INTRAMUSCULAR (I.M.)**
      (within)    (muscle)     (within the muscle)

The most common usage of **intra-** is seen in the term:

      **INTRA + VENOUS = INTRAVENOUS (I.V.)** (in"trah-ve'nus)
      (within)    (vein)        (within a vein)

You will notice the abbreviations I.M. and I.V. have been added to these two terms. Certain therapeutic drugs or solutions may either be given **I.M.** (such as a needle shot into a muscle) or **I.V.** (a needle directly into a vein).

Other examples using stems you've become familiar with include:

**INTRA/CELLULAR** (in"trah-sel'u-lar)—within a cell

**INTRA/GLANDULAR** (in"trah-glan'du-lar)—within a gland

# EXERCISE 25:

---

The stem **hepat** refers to the liver. Where would **intrahepatic** (in"trah-hĕ-pat'ik) be? _____

(Answer on page 33)

The prefix **inter-** means the opposite—situated, formed, or occurring between or among elements, as in the term **interlabial** (in″ter-la′be-al) (between the lips):

**INTER  + LABIAL  =  INTERLABIAL**
(between)     (lips)     (between the lips)

# EXERCISE 26:

Define the following terms:

1. intercellular (in″ter-sel′u-lar) _____
2. intermuscular (in″ter-mus′ku-lar) _____
3. intervascular (in″ter-vas′ku-lar) _____

(Answers on page 33)

If you still have trouble distinguishing between the two prefixes **inter-** and **intra-,** think of an interstate highway—it goes **between** or connects two or more states.

We have been discussing prefixes that mean between or within. Let's learn the prefix which means around: **peri-.** Examples are **periarthric** (per″e-ar′thrik)—around a joint; and **peritonitis** (per″e-ton-i-tis)—inflammation of the **peritoneum** (per″i-to-ne′um), the lining of the abdominal and pelvic walls.

# EXERCISE 27:

Which term describes an inflammatory disease affecting the membranous sac surrounding the heart?

a. pericarditis (per″ĭ-kar-di′tis) (page 34)
b. periadenitis (per″e-ad″e-ni′tis) (page 34)
c. periaortitis (per″e-a″or-ti′tis) (page 34)

Other common terms include:

**PERI/ODONT/ITIS** (per"e-o-don-ti'tis)—inflammation of the tissues
(around) (tooth) (inflammation)      around the teeth

**PERI/STALSIS** (per" ĭ-stal'sis)—the wormlike or wavelike movement of
(around) (contraction)          the intestines. The muscles contract to
                                create movement of the contents.

**Para- (par-)** is a prefix meaning beside, around, near, beyond, accessory to, or abnormal. Quite a varied assortment of definitions, isn't it?

Here are some terms which include this prefix:

**PARA/CARDIAC** (par"ah-kar'de-ak)—beside the heart
(beside) (heart)

**PARA/CENTESIS** (par"ah-sen-te'sis)—surgical puncture of a cavity to drain
(beyond) (puncture)          fluids

**PARA/MEDICAL** (par"ah-med'ĭ-kal)—an individual whose occupation is
(near, around) (medicine)        related very closely to the medical
                                 field (eg, social workers, physical
                                 therapists, trained ambulance
                                 drivers, etc.)

**PAR/ENTERAL** (pah-ren'ter-al)—something (usually a medication) that en-
(beside, around) (intestines)    ters the body by another avenue besides the
                                 intestines, such as I.V., I.M., or SubQ (sub-
                                 cutaneous, beneath the skin) injection.


# EXERCISE 28:

---

From what you've already learned about the stem **hepat-**, what would **parahe-patic** (par"ah-he-pat'ik) describe?

a. on top of the liver (page 34)
b. beside the liver (page 34)


Another prefix that describes location is **epi-**, meaning on, upon, over, or in addition to. Your **epidermis** (ep" ĭ-der'mis) is your outermost layer of skin. The **epi-**

**gastrium** (ep″ĭ-gas′tre-um) region is the part of the body *over* the stomach (gastr). Other terms employing this word element include:

**EPI/CONDYLUS** (ep″ĭ-kon′di-lus)—an eminence on a bone, above its condyle (also called an epicondyle)

**EPI/GLOTTIS** (ep″ĭ-glot′is)—the lidlike structure covering the opening of the larynx

# EXERCISE 29:

---

The **adrenal** (ah-dre′nal) glands are located on the surface of the kidneys. Using this clue along with other word elements you've learned, select the hormone that is secreted from the adrenal glands:

a. androgen (an′dro-jen) (page 34)
b. epinephrine (ep′ĭ-nef′rin) (page 35)
c. estrogen (es′tro-jen) (page 35)

# EXERCISE 30:

---

Where would you find the **epicardium** (ep″ĭ-kar′de-um)?_____

(Answer on page 35)

To describe backward, in back of, or behind, we use the prefix **retro-,** as in the term **retroflexed** (re″tro-flekst):

**RETR(O)  +  FLEX  +  (ED)  =  RETROFLEXED**
(back)            (bent)              (bent back)

# EXERCISE 31:

Which of the following terms describes a reverse or backward **peristaltic** (worm-like contraction of intestines) action? Meaning of the stems is **puls** (drive); **plas** (shape, formation); **stalsis** (contraction).

    a. retropulsion (re"tro-pul'shun) (page 35)
    b. retroplasia (re"tro-pla'se-ah) (page 35)
    c. retrostalsis (re"tro-stal'sis) (page 36)

Another prefix which can mean back is **re-**. It also means again or contrary. A **reaction** is an action contrary or opposite to the desired action. A **recurrence** of disease symptoms means that they have appeared again (or come back) after having disappeared for a while. A **retractor** is a surgical instrument that draws back organs or tissues and holds them out of the way during an operation.

The opposite of back is in front of or before, which is identified by several prefixes:

    **PRE**—before, in front of
    **PRO**—in front of, before, forward
    **ANTE**—before

**Ante-** is a prefix that you will encounter repeatedly. It signifies before in time or place as in the term **ante cibum** (an'te si'bum) (a.c.)—before meals. Other examples include **antecubital** (an"te-ku'bi-tal)—situated in front of or before the cubitus (forearm); **ante mortem** (an'te mor'tem)—before death; and **anterior** (an-te'-re-or)—situated in front of or in the forward part of.

# EXERCISE 32:

If we told you that the stem **febr** means fever, which of the following terms would you judge means before the onset of fever?

a. antifebrile (an"tǐ-feb'ril) (page 36)

b. antefebrile (an"te-feb'ril) (page 36)

The prefix **antero-** is used in a manner similar to the prefix **ante-**. It also means before, as in the term **anterograde** (an'ter-o-grad")—moving or extending forward.

In addition to the prefixes **ante-** and **antero-**, we find another prefix used to indicate before. This prefix is **pre-**, as in the term **preinvasive** (pre"in-va'siv)—not yet invading the tissues; **prenatal** (pre-na'tal)—existing or occurring before birth; and **preoperative** (pre-op'er-a"tiv)—preceding an operation.

# EXERCISE 33:

If we told you the meaning of **malignant** (mah-lig'nant) was related to the deadliness or worsening of disease, **morbid** (mor'bid) was related to disease or diseased, and **mortal** (mor'tal) was related to death, what should you determine to be a proper term meaning "occurring before the development of a disease?"

a. premorbid (pre-mor'bid) (page 36)

b. premortal (pre-mor'tal) (page 37)

c. premalignant (pre"mah-lig'nant) (page 37)

The third prefix **pro-** is not quite as common. Examples of its usage are:

**PROG/NOSIS** (prog-no'sis)—a forecast for the progress and outcome of a
(before) (knowledge)          disease

**PRO/LAPSE** (pro-laps')—a falling down or sinking forward of a body part
(before) (fall)

The prefix used to designate after (time) and behind (location) is **post-**. For example, **posterior** (pos-te're-or) means situated behind or toward the rear; **postoperative** (post-op'er-a"tiv) means occurring after an operation; and **postmortem** (post-mor'tem) means occurring or performed after death.

## EXERCISE 34:

Which of the following terms denotes occurrence after birth?

a.  postnatal (post-na′tal) (page 37)
b.  prenatal (pre-na′tal) (page 38)

**Per-** means through. Examples of its usage include:

**PER/FORATE** (per′fo-rāt)—to go through

**PER/MEABLE** (per′me-ah-bl)—allowing substances to pass through
(through) (to pass)

**PER OS**—by mouth

Two other prefixes which have similar meanings are **mal-** and **dys-,** both meaning bad, difficult, or painful. Examine the following terms:

**DYS/MENORRHEA** (dis″men-o-re′ah)—painful menstruation

**MAL/NUTRITION**—insufficient diet, and disorder of nutrition

**MAL/PRACTICE**—improper (bad) practice

## EXERCISE 35:

Define the following terms:

dysentery (dis′en-ter″e) _____ of the intestines
dyslexia (dis-lek′se-ah) _____ with reading
malocclusion (mal″o-kloo′zhun) _____ positioning of the teeth
dysphasia (dis-fa′ze-ah) _____ with speech
dyspnea (disp′ne-ah) _____ breathing
dysuria (dis-u′re-ah) _____ urination

(Answers on page 38)

# CHAPTER 1 ANSWERS

---

**YOUR ANSWER: 1a.** (1) beginning, (2) stem, (3) suffix

You are correct. Many medical terms involve a prefix, a stem, and a suffix—the prefix being placed at the beginning and the suffix being placed at the end of the stem, main body, or root of the word. Return to page 4.

**YOUR ANSWER: 1b.** (1) beginning, (2) prefix, (3) suffix

Almost, but not quite. If you will remember, we indicated that the stem is the main body of the word and not the prefix as you indicated. The stem of a medical term usually indicates the tissue or organ or body system which is involved in a disease process, such as derma- (skin), nephro- (kidney), and neuro- (nerve). Please return to page 4 and select the correct answer from the alternatives listed.

**YOUR ANSWER: 2a.** miscarriage

Correct. The medical term **abortion** does mean miscarriage or expulsion of the fetus before its proper time (ie, away from the normal time for a birth to occur). Return to page 5.

**YOUR ANSWER: 2b.** normal birth

You are incorrect. There is nothing in the prefix or stem of the term **abortion** which would indicate that the answer you chose might be correct. The prefix **ab-** means away from and the stem means to be born (from the Latin *oriri*). Therefore, abortion means away from being born, not born. Please return to page 5 and choose the correct answer from the alternatives listed.

**EXERCISE 3 ANSWER:**

> **DIS/LOCATION**—apart from the normal location or out of position (usu-
> (away from)      ally referring to a bone). Return to page 6.
> (location)

**YOUR ANSWER: 4a.** a muscle that moves part of the body away from the midline

This is incorrect. The prefix **ab-** indicates away from. The word **adductor** is the muscle we are asking you to define. **Ad-** means to or toward. Return to page 6 and continue.

**YOUR ANSWER:   4b.**   a muscle that brings a part of the body toward the midline

You are correct. The prefix **ad-** does indicate to or toward, making the word **adductor** mean the muscle which will move to or toward something (here, the midline of the body). Return to page 7 and go on to Exercise 5.

**YOUR ANSWER:   5a.**   near the kidneys

Correct. Adrenal means near the kidneys because the prefix **ad-** indicates to you that it is near, to, or toward the stem, no matter what root word or stem is used. Adrenal is the name of a gland on top of the kidneys. Return to page 7.

**YOUR ANSWER:   5b.**   **away from the kidneys**

Incorrect. Remember the prefix **ad-** indicates to or toward something. It could also be interpreted to mean *near* something. Return to page 7 and continue.

**YOUR ANSWER:   6a.**   near the speech center of the brain

No, **aphasia** does not describe "near the speech center." What does the prefix **a-** indicate? Return to page 8 and review the question.

**YOUR ANSWER:   6b.**   unable to speak

You are correct. **Aphasia** means unable to speak, a condition usually brought about by injury or disease to the speech center of the brain. Return to page 9.

## SPELLING EXERCISE

1. **ap**nea (ap-ne′ah)
2. **an**algesia (an″al-je′ze-ah)
3. **a**menorrhea (ah-men″o-re′ah)
4. **an**acidity (an″ah-sid′ĭ-te)

**YOUR ANSWER:   7a.**   excessively active

You are correct. **Hyperactive** means excessively active. Return to page 10.

**YOUR ANSWER:    7b.**    hardly active

This is incorrect. **Hyper-** means above, excessive, or beyond. Return to page 10 and continue.

### EXERCISE 8 ANSWERS:

1. hypoacidity    *less than normal acidity*
2. hypoglycemia    *abnormally low level of sugar in the blood*

**YOUR ANSWER:    9a.**    on the surface of the skin

This is incorrect. Above or on the surface of would be indicated by the prefix **hyper-**. Return to page 10 and choose another answer.

**YOUR ANSWER:    9b.**    beneath the skin

You are correct. A hypodermic injection would be one given under the skin. Return to page 10.

**YOUR ANSWER:    10a.**    hypothermia

You are correct. The prefix **hypo-** means low or below. Go to page 11.

**YOUR ANSWER:    10b.**    hyperthermia

You are incorrect. The prefix **hyper-** means abnormally high. Review the last few frames if you are uncertain of the definition of the two prefixes **hyper-** and **hypo-**. Return to page 11 and select another answer after reviewing the material.

### EXERCISE 11 ANSWER:

subcutaneous    *beneath the skin*

Return to page 11.

**YOUR ANSWER:    12a.**    subarcuate

You are incorrect. The term **subarcuate** means somewhat arched or bent. It is not related to the question posed, which deals with a disease process. Please return to page 12 and select the correct answer from the alternatives provided.

**YOUR ANSWER:    12b.**    subacute

You are correct. **Subacute** does mean somewhat acute—between the state of being acute and the state of being chronic. Such a condition is not quite severe enough to be called acute, nor of sufficient duration to be called chronic. Return to page 12.

**EXERCISE 13 ANSWERS:**

1. supranormal    *greater than normal, excessive amounts*
2. supra-axillary    *above the armpit*

**YOUR ANSWER:    14a.**    subpubic

Incorrect. **Subpubic** indicates the area below the pubic arch. Return to page 13 and continue.

**YOUR ANSWER:    14b.**    suprapubic

Correct. **Suprapubic** *does* indicate the region above the pubic arch. Return to page 13.

**YOUR ANSWER:    15a.**    submersion in water

Incorrect. Although the prefix **de-** means down, it does not mean that in the physical sense as does **sub-**. Return to page 13 and continue.

**YOUR ANSWER:    15b.**    removal of water

Correct. **Dehydration** is the condition in which water has been removed from a substance; usually, it refers to the excessive loss of body water. Return to page 14.

**EXERCISE 16 ANSWERS:**

1. deacidify    *taking out or removal of acid*
2. decompression    *removal or relief of pressure*
3. desensitize    *to remove sensation*
4. decontaminate    *to remove contamination such as radioactive material or bacteria*

**YOUR ANSWER:    17a.**    a condition or disease which would make the medication or treatment useless or harmful

Correct. The term contraindication means:

**CONTRA + INDICATION =    CONTRAINDICATION**
(opposing)                              (opposite of the indicated
                                                   or desired result or treatment)

Return to page 15.

**YOUR ANSWER:    17b.**    a medication given on opposite days of the week

This is incorrect. **Contra-** does mean opposite but not in the sense of every other in this term. Review the question again and select another answer from page 14.

**YOUR ANSWER:    18a.**    working together

Incorrect. The prefix **co-** indicates together but **hesive** comes from the Latin *haerere,* which means to stick; therefore, cohesive means uniting together (answer b). Particles are united together by the force called cohesion. Continue on page 15.

**YOUR ANSWER:    18b.**    uniting together

Correct. The force which causes particles or bodies to unite together is called **cohesion.** When they are uniting together, they are cohesive. Return to page 15.

**YOUR ANSWER:    19a.**    working together

Correct. **Synergy** is a coordinated effort of structures (such as muscles in movement) or drugs for therapy. Return to page 17.

**YOUR ANSWER:    19b.**    looking like work

Not exactly. Synergy not only looks like work, it *is* work—a working together. Go to page 17 and continue.

**YOUR ANSWER:    20a.**    (1) tachy (-stalsis) (2) brady (-phrenia)

You are incorrect—in fact, you have the prefixes just reversed. While the question asked for the term describing slowness in intestinal movement, you answered by choosing the prefix **tachy-** indicating fast; also, while the question asked for the term describing the rapidity of thought processes, you chose the prefix **brady-** indicating slowness. If you are confusing the two, think of a tachometer on a car or boat—it tells how *fast* you are going. Redo the question on page 17 and continue with answer b.

**YOUR ANSWER:   20b.**   (1) brady (-stalsis) (2) tachy (-phrenia)

You are correct. Bradystalsis (brad"e-stal'sis) does mean abnormally slow peristalsis—intestinal contractions; and **tachyphrenia** does mean extreme mental hyperactivity or rapidity of thought processes.

**BRADY +         STALSIS       =       BRADYSTALSIS**
(slow)      (send by contraction)    (abnormally slow peristalsis,
                                        intestinal contractions)

**TACHY    + PHREN +         IA        =       TACHYPHRENIA**
(fast, rapid)     (mind)     (condition of)    (extreme rapidity of mental
                                                        processes)

Return to page 18.

**EXERCISE 21 ANSWERS:**

1. extracardial   *outside the heart*
2. exocrine   *external (outside) secretion*
3. extracranial   *outside of the skull*
4. extubate   *removal of a tube*

**YOUR ANSWER:   22a.**   exostosis

You are incorrect. The term you chose as the correct answer—exostosis—means a bony growth projecting out from the surface of a bone.

**EX    + OS (TO) +     SIS      =       EXOSTOSIS**
(out of)     (bone)      (state or      (growth or projection
                          condition)       out from a bone)

Please return to page 19 and select the correct answer from the alternatives provided.

**YOUR ANSWER:   22b.**   exotoxin

You are correct. **Exotoxin** (ek"so-tok'sin) is the term used to describe a toxin formed by bacteria which is found outside the bacterial cell. It is in contrast to **en-**

**dotoxin** (en"do-tok'sin), which is a toxic substance found within the bacterial cell. Return to page 19.

## YOUR ANSWER:   22c.   exoserosis

You are incorrect. Exoserosis is a medical term describing the oozing of serum or exudate, as in moist skin diseases:

$$\underset{\text{(out of)}}{\textbf{EX(O)}} + \underset{\text{(serum)}}{\textbf{SERO}} + \underset{\substack{\text{(condition} \\ \text{or state of)}}}{\textbf{SIS}} = \underset{\substack{\text{(condition or state of serum} \\ \text{oozing out of)}}}{\textbf{EXOSEROSIS}}$$

Please return to page 19 and select the correct answer from the alternatives provided.

## YOUR ANSWER:   23a.   a toxin found inside the bacterial cell

Correct. **Endotoxin** is a toxic substance found *inside* a bacterial cell. Return to page 20.

## YOUR ANSWER:   23b.   a toxin found on the outer edge of a bacterial cell.

Incorrect. Remember what prefix indicates outer or outside? The term described here would be exotoxin. Return to page 20 and continue.

## EXERCISE 24 ANSWER:

endotracheal tube    *placed inside the trachea (windpipe)*

## EXERCISE 25 ANSWER:

intrahepatic    *within the liver*

## EXERCISE 26 ANSWERS:

1. intercellular    *between cells*
2. intermuscular    *between two muscles*
3. intervascular    *between blood vessels*

**YOUR ANSWER: 27a.** pericarditis

You are correct. **Pericarditis** does describe the disease in which the membranous sac that surrounds the heart, the **pericardium** (per"i-kar'de-um), becomes inflamed, as:

PERI + CARD + ITIS = PERICARDITIS

(around)  (heart)  (inflammation)  (inflammation of the membrane surrounding the heart)

Continue on page 22.

**YOUR ANSWER: 27b.** periadenitis

You are incorrect. **Periadenitis** does not describe an inflammation of the membrane surrounding the heart. Instead, the term describes inflammation of the tissues surrounding a gland. The stem **aden** refers to a gland. Please return to page 21 and select the correct answer from the alternatives listed.

**YOUR ANSWER: 27c.** periaortitis

You are incorrect. The term you chose for the answer describes a condition in which the tissues around the aorta are inflamed. Please return to page 21 and choose the correct answer from the alternatives listed.

**YOUR ANSWER: 28a.** on top of the liver

You are incorrect. The prefix **para-** indicates beside or around, not on top of. Return to page 22 and select another answer.

**YOUR ANSWER: 28b.** beside the liver

Correct. The word **parahepatic** (par"ah-he-pat'ik) means beside the liver:

PARA + HEPATIC = PARAHEPATIC

(beside)  (liver)  (beside the liver)

Return to page 22.

**YOUR ANSWER: 29a.** androgen

You are incorrect. **Androgen** is the technical term for the male sex hormone, as:

| ANDR(O) + | GEN | = | ANDROGEN |
|---|---|---|---|
| (man) | (a substance that produces or generates) | | (substance producing man[ly] characteristics) |

The term androgen is not related to the clues provided (surface and kidneys). Please return to page 23 and select another answer from the alternatives listed.

## YOUR ANSWER: 29b. epinephrine

Correct. **Epinephrine** is the name of the hormone secreted by the adrenal glands which are located on the surface of the kidneys (the derivation is epi = on or upon, plus nephr[o] = kidneys). Return to page 23.

## YOUR ANSWER: 29c. estrogen

You are incorrect. Estrogen is not related to the clues (surface and kidney) provided to help you in figuring out the answer to this question. Estrogen refers to the female sex hormone, as:

| ESTR(O) | + | GEN | = | ESTROGEN |
|---|---|---|---|---|
| (periodic changes in female reproductive organs) | | (substances that produces or generates) | | (hormone associated with reproductive system changes) |

Return to page 23 and select another alternative after reviewing the question.

## EXERCISE 30 ANSWER:

Where would you find the epicardium? *around the heart*

## YOUR ANSWER: 31a. retropulsion

You are incorrect. Retropulsion does not refer to peristaltic action. Rather, the term describes a condition of driving back, as of the fetal head during labor. Please return to page 24 and select the correct answer from the alternatives provided.

## YOUR ANSWER: 31b. retroplasia

You are incorrect. Retroplasia describes the degeneration of a tissue into a more primitive type and is not related to peristalsis, either normal or backward:

$$\underset{\text{(backward)}}{\textbf{RETRO}} + \underset{\text{(formation)}}{\textbf{PLAS(IA)}} = \underset{\substack{\text{(retrogression, degeneration} \\ \text{of tissue)}}}{\textbf{RETROPLASIA}}$$

Please return to page 24 and select the correct answer from the alternatives provided.

## YOUR ANSWER: 31c.   retrostalsis

You are correct. Retrostalsis does refer to the condition of reversed or backward peristaltic action:

$$\underset{\text{(backward)}}{\textbf{RETR(O)}} + \underset{\text{(contraction)}}{\textbf{STAL}} + \underset{\text{(state of)}}{\textbf{SIS}} = \underset{\substack{\text{(reversed peristaltic} \\ \text{[contractive] action)}}}{\textbf{RETROSTALSIS}}$$

Return to page 24.

## YOUR ANSWER: 32a.   antifebrile

You are incorrect. Antifebrile means relieving or reducing fever.

$$\underset{\substack{\text{(against;} \\ \text{counter)}}}{\textbf{ANTI}} + \underset{\text{(fever)}}{\textbf{FEBR}} + \underset{\text{(pertaining to)}}{\textbf{ILE}} = \underset{\substack{\text{(reduction, counteracting} \\ \text{a fever)}}}{\textbf{ANTIFEBRILE}}$$

Please return to page 25 and select the correct answer from the alternatives provided.

## YOUR ANSWER: 32b.   antefebrile

You are correct. Antefebrile does mean before the onset of fever. Return to page 25.

## YOUR ANSWER: 33a.   premorbid

Correct. Premorbid does indicate occurrence before the actual development of disease:

$$\underset{\text{(before)}}{\textbf{PRE}} + \underset{\text{(disease)}}{\textbf{MORBID}} = \underset{\text{(occurring before disease)}}{\textbf{PREMORBID}}$$

Return to page 25.

**YOUR ANSWER:  33b.**   premortal

You are incorrect. Your error is understandable, but premortal means occurring just before death—not just before occurrence of a disease:

> **PRE**   + **MORTAL** =       **PREMORTAL**
> (before)      (death)      (occurring just before death)

Please return to page 25 and select the correct answer from the alternatives provided.


**YOUR ANSWER:  33c.**   premalignant

You are incorrect. Premalignant means before or preceding the development of malignant (worsening) characteristics of a disease.

> **PRE**   + **MALIGNANT** =       **PREMALIGNANT**
> (before)      (worsening)       (preceding development of
>                                     malignancy, or worsening)

Please return to page 25 and select the correct answer from the answers provided.


**YOUR ANSWER:  34a.**   postnatal

You are correct. Postnatal (post-na'tal) does mean occurring after birth:

> **POST + NATAL** =       **POSTNATAL**
> (after)      (birth)      (occurring after birth)

The term postpartum (post-par'tum) also means occurring after childbirth or after delivery:

> **POST +       PARTUM**        =   **POSTPARTUM**
> (after)      (labor or childbirth)      (occurring after labor
>                                            or childbirth)

Remember, however, that the term postnatal is used in discussing conditions affecting the **neonate** (ne'o-nat) or newborn child, whereas the term postpartum refers to the mother's condition subsequent to delivery. Continue on page 26.

**YOUR ANSWER:   34b.**   prenatal

You are incorrect. Prenatal means occurring before birth, not after birth. Please return to page 26 and select the correct answer from the alternatives provided.

**EXERCISE 35 ANSWERS:**

dysentery    *pain* of the intestines

dyslexia    *difficulty* with reading

malocclusion    *bad, incorrect* positioning of the teeth

dysphasia    *difficulty* with speech

dyspnea    *difficult, painful* breathing

dysuria    *painful* urination

# CHAPTER 1 PREFIX WORD STUDY

abaxial (ab-ak′se-al)

abduction (ab-duk′shun)

abductor (ab-duk′tor)

abnormal (ab-nor′mal)

abortion (ah-bor′shun)

adaxial (ad-ak′se-al)

adduction (ah-duk′shun)

adductor (ə-duk′tər)

adhesion (ad-he′zhən)

adrenal (ah-dre′nal)

amenorrhea (ah-men″o-re′ah)

anacidity (an″ah-sid′ĭ-te)

analgesia (an″al-je′ze-ah)

anaphylaxis (an″ah-fĭ-lak′sis)

anesthesia (an″es-the′ze-ah)

ante mortem (an′te mor′tem)

ante cibum (an′te si′bum)

antecubital (an″te-ku′bi-tal)

anterograde (an′ter-o-grad″)

anterior (an-te′re-or)

antibiotic (an″tĭ-bi-ot′ik)

antipyretic (an″tĭ-pi-ret′ik)

antiseptic (an″tĭ-sep′tik)

aphasia (ah-fa′ze-ah)

apnea (ap-ne′ah)

asepsis (a-sep′sis)

assimilation (ah-sim″i-la′shun)

bradycardia (brad″e-kar′de-ah)

bradypnea (brad″e-ne′-ah)

cardiopulmonary (kar″de-o-pul′-
mo-ner-e)

cohesive (ko-he′siv)

concentrate (kon′sən-trāt)

confluent (kon′floo-ənt)

congenital (kən-jen′ĭ-təl)

constriction (kən-strik′shən)

contraception (kon″trə-sep′shən)

contraindication (kon″trah-in″-
dĭ-ka′shun)

contralateral (kon″trə-lat′ər-əl)

deacidify (de″ah-sid′ĭ-fi)

decomposition (de″kom-pə-zish′ən)

decompression (de″kom-presh′un)

decongestant (de″kən-jes′tənt)

decontaminate (de′kən-tam′a-nat′)

degerm (de-germ′)

dehydration (de″hi-dra′shun)

desensitize (de-sen′sĭ-tīz)

disability (dis″ə-bil′ĭ-te)

disinfection (dis″in-fek′shən)

dislocation (dis″lo-ka′shən)

dysentery (dis′en-ter″e)

dyslexia (dis-lek′se-ah)

dysmenorrhea (dis-men″ə-re′ə)

dysphasia (dis-fa′ze-ah)

dyspnea (disp′ne-ah)

dysuria (dis-u′re-ah)

eccentric (ek-sen′trik)

ectoderm (ek′to-dərm)

elimination (e-lim″ĭ-na′shən)

endocellular (en″do cel′u lər)

endoderm (en′do-dərm)

endotoxin (en″do-tok′sin)

endotracheal (en″do-tra′ke-al)

epicardium (ep″ĭ-kar′de-um)

epicondylus (ep″ĭ-kon″də-ləs)

epidermis (ep″ĭ-der′mis)

epigastrium (ep″ĭ-gas′tre-um)

epiglottis (ep″ĭ-glot′is)

exocrine (ek′so-krin)

expectoration (ek-spek″təra′shən)

extracardial (eks″trah-kar′de-al)

extracellular (eks″trə-sel′u-lər)

extracranial (eks″trah-kra′ne-al)

extubate (eks-tu′bāt)

hyperactive (hi″pər-ak-tiv′)

hyperglycemia (hi″per-gli-se′me-ah)

hypodermic (hi″po-der′mik)

hypoglycemia (hi″po-gli-se′me-ah)

ileum (il′e-um)

ilium (il′e-um)

intercellular (in″ter-sel′u-lar)

interlabial (in″ter-la′be-al)

intermuscular (in″ter-mus′ku-lar)

intervascular (in″ter-vas′ku-lar)

intracellular (in″trə-sel′u-lər)

intraglandular (in″trə-glan′du-lər)

intrahepatic (in″trah-hĕ-pat′ik)

intramuscular (I.M.) (in″trah-mus′-ku-lar)

intravenous (I.V.) (in″trə-ve′nəs)

malignant (mah-lig′nant)

malnutrition (mal″noo-trish′ən)

malocclusion (mal″o-kloo′zhun)

malpractice (mal-prak′tis)

morbid (mor′bid)

mortal (mor′tal)

paracardiac (par″ə-kahr′de-ak)

paracentesis (par″ə-sən-te′sis)

parahepatic (par″ah-he-pat′ik)

paramedical (par″ə-med′i-kəl)

parenteral (pə-ren′tər-əl)

perforate (per′fə-rāt″)

periarthric (per″e-ar′thrik)

periodontitis (per″e-odon-ti′tis)

peristalsis (per″ĭ-stal-sis)

peritonitis (per″ĕ-ton-i-tis)

permeable (per′me-ə-bəl)

per os (p.o.) (pər os)

posterior (pos-te′re-or)

postmortem (post-mor′tem)

postoperative (post-op′er-a″tiv)

prefix

preinvasive (pre″in-va′siv)

prenatal (pre-na′tal)

preoperative (pre-op′er-a″tiv)

prognosis (prog-no′sis)

prolapse (pro-laps′)

reaction (re-ak′shən)

recurrence (re-kur′əns)

retractor (re-trak′tor)

retroflexed (re″tro-flekst)

stem

subaural (səb-aw′rəl)

subaxillary (sub-ak′si-ler″e)

sublingual (sub-ling′gwal)

subnasal (səb-na′zəl)

suffix

superacute (soo″per-ah-kūt)

superlethal (soo″per-le′thal)

supra-axillary (soo″prah-ak′sĭ-ler″e)

supranormal (soo″prah-nor′məl)

symmetry (sim′ə-tre)

synarthrosis (sin″ahr-thro′sis)

syndrome (sin′drōm)

synergy (sin′er-je)

synovial (sĭ-no′ve-al)

tachycardia (tak″e-kar′de-ah)

tachypnea (tak″ip-ne′ah)

# Prefixes That Deal with Sizes and Numbers

*You have learned a lot of prefixes already but there are a few more that you need to learn. These can be classified as those prefixes which identify size and number or amount.*

## PREFIX STUDY LIST

| | | |
|---|---|---|
| alb- | leuk- | poly- |
| ambi- (amb-) | macro- | sclero- |
| bi- | mega-, megal- | semi- |
| di- | micro- | tetra-, quad- |
| hemi- | mono- | trans- |
| hetero- | multi- | tri- |
| homo- | ob- (oc-) | uni- |
| infra- | | |

Many of these prefixes should be easy to learn since they mean the same in our everyday English as they do in medical terminology.

Two prefixes mean one. They are **mono-** and **uni-**. Examples include **monocular** (mon-ok′u-lar)—having one eye, and **unilateral** (u″nĭ-lat′er-al)—affecting one side.

The prefix that means two is **bi-,** as in **biceps** (bi′seps)—a muscle with two heads. Another prefix which means two or twice is **di-,** as in the term **diphasic** (di-fa′zik)—two phases or stages.

The number three is identified by using the prefix **tri-:** think of a triangle, which has three corners. A **tricep** is a muscle that has _____ heads, and a **tricuspid** (tri-kus′pid) is a valve which has _____ connections.

To distinguish four, the prefixes **tetra-** and **quad-** are used. **Tetrameric** (tet″rah-mer′ik) means having four parts; **quadriplegia** (kwod″rĕ-ple′je-ah) means a paralysis of all four limbs.

Two prefixes that deal with an unspecified quantity are **poly-** and **multi-**. They mean much or many but are not definitive enough to tell you a specific number. Medical terms which use these include:

> **POLY/URIA** (pol″e-u′re-ah)—an abnormally large amount of urine excreted
>
> **MULTI/GRAVIDA** (mul″tĭ-grav′ĭ-dah)—a woman who has been pregnant several times
>
> **MULTI/ARTICULAR** (mul″te-ar-tik′u-lar)—affecting or pertaining to many joints
>
> **POLY/GLANDULAR** (pol″e-glan′du-lar)—pertaining to several glands

It may be difficult to decide which prefix to use when you're the one doing the word building. Here again, it's best to learn the words as a whole.

## EXERCISE 1:

Fill in the proper prefix:

1. _____ chromatic (having only one color)
2. _____ chromatic (having or able to distinguish three colors)
3. _____ chromatism (showing two colors)
4. _____ chromic (having or able to distinguish only four colors)

(Answer on page 45)

A prefix that signifies one-half is **hemi-**. You will see it in words such as **hemiplegia** (hem″e-ple′je-ah)—paralysis of one-half of the body or **hemigastrectomy** (hem″e-gas-trek′to-me)—removal of one-half of the stomach.

# EXERCISE 2:

**Opic** refers to the eye. What would **hemiopic** (hem″e-op′ik) describe?

a. affecting both eyes (page 45)
b. affecting one eye (page 45)

A similar prefix is **semi-**. **Semi-** can mean either half or partly. The **semicircular canals** in the ear are not full circles, but partially circular in shape. The **semilunar valves** found in the aorta of the heart and the pulmonary (lung) arteries are half-moon shaped.

# EXERCISE 3:

How would you describe someone in a **semicoma?**

a. able to be partially awakened from their coma (page 45)
b. totally unaware of their surroundings (page 45)

Prefixes that indicate size include **mega- (megal-)** and **macro-,** meaning large, and **micro-,** meaning small. Below are some examples of their usage.

**MEGA/BLADDER**—permanently oversized bladder
**MEGALO/CEPHALY** (meg″ah-lo-sef′ah-le)—an unusually large head size
**MACRO/CYST**—a large cyst

**MICRO/BIOLOGY**—the study of microorganisms (minute living organisms)

**MICRO/SURGERY**—surgery performed using a microscope

In medical terminology there are some words that cannot be classified as either a prefix, suffix, or root word. These words are called **combining forms.** Combining forms may appear at the beginning or in the middle of the word. They may be only a single letter added to make the word flow better in speech, for instance the **o** in **pneumorrhagia** (nu"mo-ra'je-ah)—hemorrhage from the lungs.

**Alb-** and **leuk-** are considered combining forms. They both mean white. Words that use these forms are:

**ALBUMIN** (al-bu'min)—a whitish-colored protein

**LEUKEMIA** (loo-ke'me-ah)—an abnormal condition involving the white blood cells

A few additional prefixes that you may need to know appear below along with examples of each.

| PREFIX | MEANING | EXAMPLE |
|--------|---------|---------|
| **ambi- (amb-)** | both | **AMBIDEXTROUS**—equal dexterity (ability) with both hands |
| **hetero-** | other | **HETEROSEXUAL**—pertaining to the other (opposite) sex |
| **homo-** | the same, common | **HOMOCENTRIC**—having the same center or focus |
| **infra-** | beneath | **INFRACOSTAL**—beneath a rib or ribs |
| **ob-** (**oc-** before words that begin with **c**) | against, in front of, towards (closed) | **OCCLUSION**—an obstruction or closing off, as in front of the teeth |
| **sclero-** | hard | **ARTERIOSCLEROSIS** (ar-te"re-o-skle-ro'sis)—hardening of the arteries |
| **trans-** | across, over | **TRANSECTION**—incision across the long axis; a cross section |

You may sometimes find that an individual's preference is all that decides which prefix to place before a word. Take, for instance, the terms **subcostal** and **infracostal.** Both mean beneath or below the ribs and can be used interchangeably. It just may depend on whatever the health care associate is accustomed to using. After working the exercise on page 47, continue with UNIT II, Suffixes.

# CHAPTER 2 ANSWERS

## EXERCISE 1 ANSWERS:

1. *mono*chromatic (having only one color)
2. *tri*chromatic (having or able to distinguish three colors)
3. *di*chromatism (showing two colors)
4. *tetra*chromic (having or able to distinguish only four colors)

**YOUR ANSWER:   2a.**   affecting both eyes

Incorrect. Keep in mind that **hemi-** means one-half. Since the norm is for two eyes, hemiopic would be something that affected one-half or only one eye. Continue on page 43.

**YOUR ANSWER:   2b.**   affecting one eye

Correct. Hemiopic refers to something that only affects one eye. Return to page 43.

**YOUR ANSWER:   3a.**   able to be partially awakened from their coma

You are correct. Someone in a **semicoma** is not in a full coma, but only a partial one. Return to page 43.

**YOUR ANSWER:   3b.**   totally unaware of their surroundings

Incorrect. Someone who is fully unaware of their surroundings would not fit the description of being in a semicoma. Remember that the prefix **semi-** means half or partly. Return to page 43 and continue after selecting another answer.

# CHAPTER 2 PREFIX WORD STUDY LIST

albumin (al-bu′min)

ambidextrous (am″bĭ-dek′strəs)

arteriosclerosis (ar-te″re-o-skle-ro′sis)

biceps (bi′seps)

diphasic (di-fa′zik)

hemigastrectomy (hem″e-gas-trek′
  to-me)

hemiopic (hem″e-op′ik)

hemiplegia (hem″e-ple′je-ah)

heterosexual (het″ər-o-sek′shoo-əl)

homocentric (ho″mo-sen′trik)

infracostal (in″frə-kos′təl)

leukemia (loo-ke′me-ah)

macrocyst (mak′ro-sist)

megabladder (məg″ə-blad′ər)

megalocephaly (meg″ə-lo-sef′ə-le)

microbiology (mi″kro-bi-ol′ə-je)

microsurgery (mi′kro-sər″jər-e)

monocular (mon-ok′u-lar)

multiarticular (mul″te-ahr-tik′u-lər)

multigravida (mul″tĭ-grav′ĭ-də)

occlusion (o-kloo′zhən)

polyglandular (pol″e-glan′du-lər)

polyuria (pol″e-u′re-ə)

quadriplegia (kwod″rĕ-ple′je-ah)

semicircular canals

semicoma (sem″e-ko′mə)

semilunar (sem″-e-loo-nər) valves

tetrameric (tet″rah-mer′ik)

transection (tran-sek′-shən)

tricep (tri′sep)

tricuspid (tri-kus′pid)

unilateral (u″nĭ-lat′er-al)

## PREFIX EXERCISE

Match the following prefixes from Column A with the definitions in Column B. Some definitions may be used more than once.

**A**

1. a- _____
2. endo- _____
3. anti- _____
4. hypo- _____
5. tachy- _____
6. mal- _____
7. intra- _____
8. ante- _____
9. hyper- _____
10. exo- _____
11. epi- _____
12. retro- _____
13. dys- _____
14. inter- _____
15. an- _____

**B**

A. slow

B. between

C. above, excessive

D. without, not

E. bad

F. within, inside

G. backwards

H. on, upon

I. before

J. together

K. below, beneath

L. fast

M. near

N. against

O. out, away from

(Answers in Appendix on page 259.)

# PREFIX PUZZLE

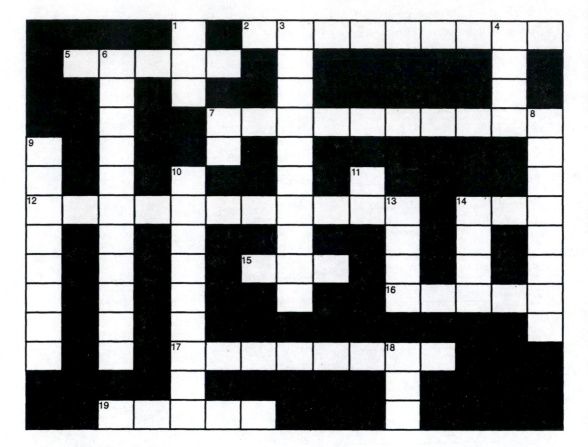

## CLUES FOR PREFIX PUZZLE

### Across

2. Large cyst
5. Prefix for small
7. Without sensation or feeling
12. Rapid heartbeat
14. Prefix meaning before
15. Prefix meaning through
16. Prefix meaning within
17. A group of symptoms which occur together
19. Prefix meaning through

## Down

1. Prefix meaning three
3. Before death
4. Prefix meaning half or partly
6. Between the ribs
7. Prefix meaning to, toward
8. Away from the norm
9. In front of
10. Difficulty with speech
11. Prefix meaning two
13. Prefix meaning against
14. Prefix meaning after
18. Prefix for bad

(Answers on page 260.)

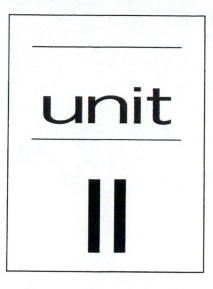

# unit

# II

# SUFFIXES

## 3: Diagnostic and Symptomatic Suffixes

Suffixes that help identify the patient's diagnosis or symptoms or condition from which he or she is suffering.

## 4: Surgical Suffixes

Suffixes that describe the type of operative procedure to be performed.

II

# chapter three

# Diagnostic and Symptomatic Suffixes

*This unit will cover suffixes—elements attached to the end of a word to further its meaning. Many of the same roots used with prefixes in Unit I will be found in Unit II. This first chapter covers suffixes that help describe the patient's condition or the diagnosis of the patient's problem. These suffixes are added to the stem or root word, which is usually descriptive of the area of the body where the problem occurs.*

## SUFFIX STUDY LIST

| | | |
|---|---|---|
| -algia | -itis | -osis |
| -cele | -lysis | -pathy |
| -emia | -logy | -penia |
| -ectasis | -malacia | -ptosis |
| -form | -megaly | -rrhage |
| -genic | -oid | -rhexis |
| -gram, graph | -ia | -spasm |
| -iasis | -oma | |

The suffix **-algia,** meaning pain, can be placed after the stem for nerve (**neur-**) to give us the word **neuralgia** (nu-ral'je-ah), which means pain along one or more nerves. You previously learned that the stem **nephr-** referred to the kidneys. Write the word that would mean kidney pain: _____ (see page 63 for answer).

The suffix **-itis** means inflammation. If we were to talk about **nephritis** (nə-fri'tis), it would mean an inflammation of _____ (see page 63 for answer). This condition could be painful and cause nephralgia. **-Itis** is a diagnostic suffix that you will see frequently; together with a stem, it describes the part of the body that is inflamed.

# EXERCISE 1:

Using stems with which you're already familiar, define the following terms:

1. phlebitis (fle-bi'tis) _____ of a vein
2. carditis (kar-di'tis) inflammation of the _____
3. arteritis (ar″tĕ-ri'tis) _____ of an artery

(Answers on page 63)

# EXERCISE 2:

Which of the following terms describes (1) a painful joint and (2) an inflamed joint?

a. (1) arthritis (ar-thri'tis)      (2) arthralgia (ar-thral'je-ah) (page 63)
b. (1) arteralgia (ar″ter-al'je-ah)   (2) arteritis (ar″tĕ-ri'tis) (page 63)
c. (1) arthralgia (ar-thral'je-ah)   (2) arthritis (ar-thri'tis) (page 63)

A suffix which means a protrusion, tumor, or swelling is **-cele.** In the term **gastrocele** (gas'tro-sēl), we are describing a hernia of the stomach (gastr). **Myelocele**

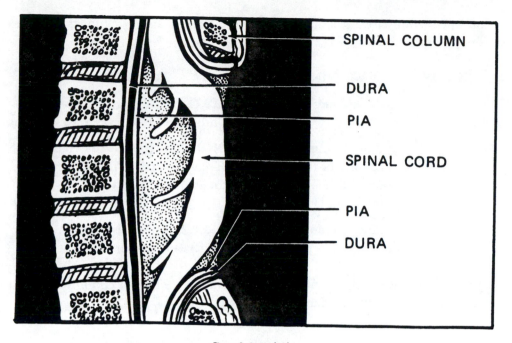

**Figure 3–1.** Myelocele

(mi-el′o-sēl) describes a protrusion of the spinal cord (myelo) through a defect in the vertebrae (see Fig. 3–1).

# EXERCISE 3:

A **cyst** is any fluid-filled sac but most often refers to the urinary bladder. Which word describes a hernia of the bladder?

a. cystocele (sis′to-sēl) (page 63)
b. cystitis (sis-ti′tis) (page 64)
c. cystalgia (sis-tal′je-ah) (page 64)

You will encounter three suffixes that have similar meanings. Study the suffixes and examples given below:

| SUFFIX | MEANING | EXAMPLE |
|--------|---------|---------|
| -ia | a state or condition | **BRADYCARDIA** (brad"e-kar'de-ah)— condition of having a slow heartbeat |
| -iasis | condition, formation of, presence of (usually used with the element lith- [stone]) | **NEPHROLITHIASIS** (nef"ro-li-thi'-ah-sis)—the presence of kidney stones |
| -osis | condition, abnormal increase of a disease | **NEUROSIS** (nu-ro'sis)—disorder of the nervous system |

You can see that the three suffixes are interrelated. They all could be defined as "condition of," but they each have distinct meanings.


# EXERCISE 4:

Keeping in mind that **derma-** referred to skin, what would the term **dermatosis** (der"mah-to'sis) mean?

a. the decline of a skin disease (page 64)
b. any condition of the skin (page 64)


# EXERCISE 5:

**Pneumonia** could best be defined as:

a. pain in the lungs (page 64)
b. a state of the lungs (page 64)

## BONUS BRAIN TEASER:

What other word would also describe inflammation of the lungs? _____
(answer on page 64)

The suffix that is used to describe the origin of a disease or medical problem is
**-genic,** which also means producing. Let's look at several examples:

> **NEUR(O)** +   **-GENIC**   =  **NEUROGENIC** (nu″ro-jen′ik)
>   (nerve)      (origin)        (originating in the nerves)

> **OSTEO-** +   **-GENIC**   =  **OSTEOGENIC** (os″te-o-jen′ik)
>   (bone)      (origin)       (originating in the bones)

> **PATH(O)** +   **-GENIC**   =  **PATHOGENIC** (path-o-jen′ik)
>   (disease)   (producing,       (disease producing)
>          originating)

## EXERCISE 6:

**Cyto-** means cell. What would **cytogenic** (si-to-jen′ik) refer to?

a. the development of cells (page 64)
b. a disease of the cells (page 65)

You were just introduced to the stem **path** in the word **pathogenic.** It also forms
part of the suffix **-pathy,** referring to disease. **Myopathy** (mi-op′ah-the) is any disease
of a muscle; similarly, **neuropathy** (nu-rop′ah-the) is a general term used to describe
disorders of the nervous system.

# EXERCISE 7:

Remember that **myelo-** referred to the spinal cord? How would you describe the general term for any disease or disorders of the spinal cord?

a. myelosis (mi″ĕ-lo′sis) (page 65)
b. myelopathy (mi″ĕ-lop′ah-the) (page 65)

The suffix for a condition involving blood is **-emia.** The term **anemia** (ah-ne′me-ah) literally means without blood, as:

$$\underset{\text{(without)}}{\textbf{AN-}} + \underset{\text{(blood)}}{\textbf{-EMIA}} = \underset{\substack{\text{(reduced number of} \\ \text{red corpuscles)}}}{\textbf{ANEMIA}}$$

Septicemia (sep″ti-se′me-ah) is a medical term meaning blood poisoning, as:

$$\underset{\text{(poison)}}{\textbf{SEPTIC-}} + \underset{\text{(blood)}}{\textbf{-EMIA}} = \underset{\text{(blood poisoning)}}{\textbf{SEPTICEMIA}}$$

Pyemia (pi-e′me-ah) also means blood poisoning characterized by the formation of pus:

$$\underset{\text{(pus)}}{\textbf{PY-}} + \underset{\text{(blood)}}{\textbf{-EMIA}} = \underset{\text{(generalized septicemia)}}{\textbf{PYEMIA}}$$

Two other suffixes that are similar are **-rhexis** (rupture) and **-rrhage** (excessive flow). **-Rhexis** refers to a more sudden rupture of an organ or vessel than does **-rrhage,** which means there is an excessive flow or discharge but not necessarily occurring suddenly, although it can. The term **hemorrhage** (hem′or-ij) means there is an excessive flow of blood (hemo). **Enterorrhexis** (en″ter-o-rek′sis) means a rupture of the intestines.

## EXERCISE 8:

_____

From what you just learned, what would the term cardiorrhexis

(kar"de-o-rek'sis) mean? _____

pneumorrhagia (nu"mo-ra'je-ah)? _____

(Answers on page 65)

## EXERCISE 9:

_____

What would you say the medical term **leukemia** (lu-ke'me-ah) describes?

a. a condition involving the white blood cells (page 65)
b. albumin in the urine (page 65)

You learned in Unit I that the prefix **mega(l)-** means large. The _suffix_ that refers to an enlarged condition is **-megaly.** Examples of this are:

**ACRO/MEGALY** (ak"ro-meg'ah-le)—a disease condition in which certain
(extreme, extremity)                    extremities of the body are enlarged,
   (enlargement)                        such as the fingers, toes, nose
**SPLENO/MEGALY** (sple"no-meg'ah-le)—enlargement of the spleen
(spleen)  (enlargement)

## EXERCISE 10:

_____

Define the following terms:

nephromegaly (nef"ro-meg'ah-le) _____
cardiomegaly (kar"de-o-meg'ah-le) _____
hepatomegaly (hep"ah-to-meg'ah-le) _____

(Answers on page 66)

The suffix that describes a tumor or swelling is **-oma.** You will see the suffix frequently if studying **oncology** (ong-kol′o-je)—cancer patients. A term that is used to describe a malignant cancer or growth of cells is **carcinoma** (kar″sĭ-no′mah). An **adenoma** (ad″ĕ-no′mah) is any glandular tumor (aden = gland).

# EXERCISE 11:

---

If an osteoma (os″te-o′mah) is a tumor composed of bony tissue, what would a **nephroma** (nĕ-fro′mah) be?

    a.  a tumor composed of nerve tissue (page 66)
    b.  a tumor composed of kidney tissue (page 66)

The suffix that denotes the process of loosening, breaking down, or dissolving is **-lysis** (li′sis). Examples include **hemolysis** (he-mol′ĭ-sis)—the breaking down or separating of hemoglobin from the red blood cells, and **myolysis** (mi-ol′ĭ-sis)—the destruction of muscular tissue.

If one body part becomes abnormally attached to another because of adhesions, the term **-lysis** may be used to describe the process for loosening the two parts, as in **gastrolysis** (gas-trol′ĭ-sis)—the loosening of the stomach from adhesions.

# EXERCISE 12:

---

Following this train of thought, what would the term **cardiolysis** (kar″de-ol′ĭ-sis) describe?

    a.  the freeing of the heart from adhesions (page 66)
    b.  the freeing of cancerous tumors from adhesions (page 66)

The dissolution or breaking down process may either be surgical or chemical. In the case of **neurolysis** (nu-rol'ĭ-sis), it describes the surgical cutting of the nerve to free it.

The word element **lysis** (li'sis) may also be used by itself, without being attached to a stem, eg, the notation on a surgery schedule—"lysis of adhesions." In this instance, the term may also refer to the gradual decline of a disease and its symptoms (as opposed to crisis, an immediate increase in disease symptoms).

To identify something as being like or resembling, the suffix **-oid** is used. A **fibroid** (fi'broid) is a tumor that resembles fibers; likewise, **sternoid** (ster'noid) refers to something that looks like the sternum (breastbone).

# EXERCISE 13:

1. What term describes something that is like lymph? _____
2. **Lip-** refers to fat. What would lipoid (lip'oid) mean? _____

(Answers on page 66)

**-Penia** is the suffix which means an abnormal deficiency or decrease. It is seen in words such as **erythropenia** (ĕ-rith"ro-pe'ne-ah)—a deficient number of erythrocytes or red blood cells in the blood, or **leukopenia** (loo"ko-pe'ne-ah)—a lack of leukocytes or white blood cells.

Other diagnostic or symptomatic suffixes that you may encounter include:

| SUFFIX | MEANING | EXAMPLE |
|---|---|---|
| **-ectasis** | expansion, dilation | **BRONCHIECTASIS** (brong"ke-ek'tah-sis) —abnormal dilatation (stretching) of bronchi |
| **-malacia** | softening | **OSTEOMALACIA** (os"te-o-mah-la'-she-ah)—softening of the bones |
| **-ptosis** | falling | **NEPHROPTOSIS** (nef"rop-to'sis)—downward displacement of the kidney |
| **-spasm** | involuntary contractions | **ENTEROSPASM** (en'ter-o-spazm)—painful intestinal contractions |

## MISCELLANEOUS WORD ENDINGS

As with prefixes, there are a few word endings that do not fit into a specific category:

| SUFFIX | MEANING | EXAMPLE |
| --- | --- | --- |
| -form | shape | DEFORMED—not normal in shape |
| -gram, -graph | a written record | ELECTROCARDIOGRAM (EKG or ECG) (e-lek"tro-kahr'de-o-gram")—a written record of the electrical activity of the heart |
| -logy | study of | BIOLOGY—the science of life and living organisms |

## EXERCISE 14:

Previously you learned what the prefix **poly-** means. What would a **polygraph** measure or record?

   a. the activity of the nervous system (page 66)
   b. the activity of several body functions (page 67)

## EXERCISE 15:

What would **cardiology** describe? _____

(Answer on page 67)

Continue with Chapter 4, Surgical Suffixes.

**PAGE 54:**

kidney pain    *nephralgia*
nephritis    inflammation of a *kidney*

**EXERCISE 1 ANSWERS:**

1. phlebitis    *inflammation* of a vein
2. carditis    inflammation of the *heart*
3. arteritis    *inflammation* of an artery

**YOUR ANSWER:    2a.**    (1) arthritis and (2) arthralgia

Incorrect. You have the two terms reversed. Remember again that **-itis** means inflamed and **-algia** refers to pain (which *may* be caused by the inflammation but not necessarily so). Keeping this in mind, return to page 54 and select another answer.

**YOUR ANSWER:    2b.**    (1) arteralgia and (2) arteritis

You are incorrect. The stem arter refers to arteries, not joints. You are correct in your usage of the suffixes **-algia** and **-itis,** however. Return to page 54 and select another answer.

**YOUR ANSWER:    2c.**    (1) arthralgia and (2) arthritis

You are correct. Arthralgia describes a painful joint and arthritis describes an inflammation of a joint. Return to page 54.

**YOUR ANSWER:    3a.**    cystocele

Correct. A **cystocele** does describe a hernia of the bladder.

|  |  |  |  |  |
|---|---|---|---|---|
| **CYST(O)-** | + | **-CELE** | = | **CYSTOCELE** |
| (bladder, fluid-filled sac) |  | (hernia, protrusion) |  | (protrusion of the bladder through the vaginal wall) |

Return to page 56.

**YOUR ANSWER:**   **3b.**   cystitis

Incorrect. Although an inflammation (**-itis**) may cause the protrusion and swelling, it does not describe the protrusion itself. Return to the question on page 55 and pick another answer.

**YOUR ANSWER:**   **3c.**   cystalgia

Incorrect. Cystalgia describes pain (**-algia**) in the bladder. The pain could be caused by the protrusion but the word **cystalgia** does not properly identify the protrusion. Return to page 55 and select a different answer.

**YOUR ANSWER:**   **4a.**   the decline of a skin disease

This is incorrect. The suffix **-osis** means condition or *increase* of a disease. Return to page 56 and continue with a different selection.

**YOUR ANSWER:**   **4b.**   any condition of the skin

Correct. Dermatosis refers to any skin condition. Return to page 56.

**YOUR ANSWER:**   **5a.**   a pain in the lungs

This is incorrect. What is the suffix that describes pain? If you remember, it is **-algia.** Look again at the word pneumonia to see what the suffix is and try again on page 56.

**YOUR ANSWER:**   **5b.**   a state of the lungs

Correct. Pneumonia is a state or condition of the lungs, specifically an infection of the lungs. Return to page 57.

## BONUS BRAIN TEASER, PAGE 57:

**Pneumonitis** would also describe inflammation of the lungs. The terms **pneumonia** and **pneumonitis** are sometimes used interchangeably, although pneumonia indicates a condition in which the lungs start to become solid or filled with secretions.

**YOUR ANSWER:**   **6a.**   the development of cells

You are correct. The word cytogenic is broken down as follows:

CYT(O)- + -GENIC =       **CYTOGENIC**
(cell)       (origin)              (the origin or
                                    development of cells)

Return to page 57.

**YOUR ANSWER:   6b.**   a disease of the cells

Incorrect. Cytogenic does not refer to a cell disease. Review the material on page 57 and answer the question again.

**YOUR ANSWER:   7a.**   myelosis

This is not correct. Myelosis is a specific condition involving the spinal cord. Myelopathy is a more general term that encompasses any disorder of the spinal cord. Continue on page 58.

**YOUR ANSWER:   7b.**   myelopathy

Correct. Myelopathy is the general term meaning any disease or disorder of the spinal cord. Return to page 58.

**EXERCISE 8 ANSWERS:**

cardiorrhexis   *rupture of the heart*
pneumorrhagia   *hemorrhage from the lungs*

**YOUR ANSWER:   9a.**   a condition involving the white blood cells

You are correct. Leukemia is a cancerous condition of the blood, involving a white cell count that is often as high as 25 times the normal value. Return to page 59.

**YOUR ANSWER:   9b.**   albumin in the urine

You are incorrect. The medical term for albumin in the urine is **albuminuria.** We are not discussing the urine at this time. The word element **leuk-** refers to white. You know that **-emia** refers to the blood, so put them together and select the correct answer from the alternatives listed on page 59.

## EXERCISE 10 ANSWERS:

nephromegaly    *enlargement of the kidney*
cardiomegaly    *an enlarged heart*
hepatomegaly    *an enlarged liver*


**YOUR ANSWER:    11a.**    a tumor composed of nerve tissue

You are incorrect. The stem **neur** would be used to describe a tumor composed of nerve tissue. The stem **nephr** means kidney; thus, a nephroma is a tumor composed of kidney tissue. Continue on page 60.


**YOUR ANSWER:    11b.**    a tumor composed of kidney tissue

Correct. A **nephroma** is a tumor composed of kidney tissue. Return to page 60.


**YOUR ANSWER:    12a.**    the freeing of the heart from adhesions

You are correct. **Cardiolysis** is the freeing of the heart from adhesions to the sternal periosteum (lining around the breastbone):

$$\text{CARDI(O)-} + \text{-LYSIS} = \text{CARDIOLYSIS}$$
$$\text{(heart)} \quad \text{(dissolution)} \quad \text{(dissolution of the heart}$$
$$\text{from its adhesions)}$$

Return to page 61.


**YOUR ANSWER:    12b.**    the freeing of cancerous tumors from adhesions

You are incorrect. Remember that the stem **cardi(o)** means heart. Try again on page 60.


## EXERCISE 13 ANSWERS:

1. Something that is like lymph is *lymphoid*
2. Lipoid means *resembling fat*


**YOUR ANSWER:    14 a.**    the activity of the nervous system

Incorrect. Remember that the prefix **poly-** means many or much. Look at the answers again on page 62 and continue.

**YOUR ANSWER:   14b.**    the activity of several body functions

Correct. **Poly-** means many or much. In this case, it also means several. A polygraph measures such things as respiratory movements, pulse, blood pressure, etc., all at the same time. Return to the exercise on page 62.

## EXERCISE 15 ANSWER:

Cardiology describes *the science and study of the heart.*

# CHAPTER 3 SUFFIX WORD STUDY LIST

acromegaly (ak″ro-meg′ə-le)

adenoma (ad″ĕ-no′mah)

anemia (ah-ne′me-ah)

arteritis (ar″tĕ-ri′tis)

biology (bi-ol′əje)

bradycardia (brad″e-kar′de-ah)

bronchiectasis (brong″ke-ek′tah-sis)

carcinoma (kar″sĭ-no′mah)

cardiology (kahr″de-ol′əje)

cardiolysis (kar″de-ol′ĭ-sis)

cardiomegaly (kar″de-o-meg′ah-le)

cardiorrhexis (kar″de-o-rek′sis)

carditis (kar-di′tis)

cyst (sist)

cytogenic (si-to-jen′ik)

deformed (de-form′d)

dermatosis (der″mah-to′sis)

electrocardiogram (e-lek″tro-kahr′de-o-
gram″)

enterorrhexis (en″ter-o-rek′sis)

enterospasm (en′ter-o-spazm)

erythropenia (ĕ-rith″ro-pe′ne-ah)

fibroid (fi′broid)

gastrocele (gas′tro-sel)

gastrolysis (gas-trol′ĭ-sis)

hemolysis (he-mol′ĭ-sis)

hemorrhage (hem′or-ij)

hepatomegaly (hep″ah-to-meg′ah-le)

leukemia (lu-ke′me-ah)

leukopenia (loo″ko-pe′ne-ah)

myelocele (mi-el′o-sel)

myolysis (mi-ol′ĭ-sis)

myopathy (mi-op′ah-the)

nephritis (nə-fri′tis)

nephrolithiasis (nef″ro-li-thi′ah-sis)

nephroma (nĕ-fro′mah)

nephromegaly (nef″ro-meg′ah-le)

nephroptosis (nef″rop-to′sis)

neuralgia (nu-ral′je-ah)

neurogenic (nu″ro-jen′ik)

neurolysis (nu-rol′ĭ-sis)

neuropathy (nu-rop′ah-the)

neurosis (nu-ro′sis)

oncology (ong-kol′o-je)

osteogenic (os″te-o-jen′ik)

osteomalacia (os″te-o-mah-la′she-ah)

pathogenic (path-o-jen′ik)

phlebitis (fle-bi′tis)

pneumonia (noo-mo-ne-ə)

pneumorrhagia (nu″mo-ra′je-ah)

polygraph (pol′e-graf)

pyemia (pi-e′me-ah)

septicemia (sep″ti-se′me-ah)

splenomegaly (sple″no-meg′ə-le)

sternoid (sternoid)

suffix

# chapter four

# Surgical Suffixes

*In our discussion, we will study the suffixes below that describe surgical procedures. You will find a diagram (Figure 4–1) of surgical locations of the body and the terms describing them to assist you in your study.*

## SUFFIX STUDY LIST

| | | |
|---|---|---|
| -centesis | -pexy | -scopy |
| -ectomy | -plasty | -(o)stomy |
| -desis | -raphy | -(o)tomy |
| -lithotomy | -sect | -tripsy |

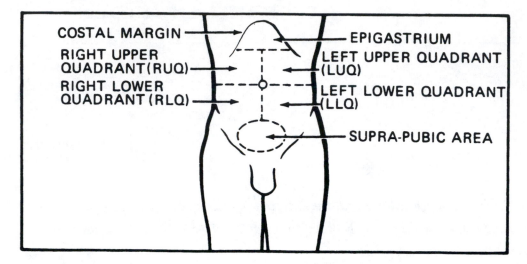

**Figure 4–1.** Surgical areas of the abdomen

Surgical suffixes are those which describe the type of surgical procedure being done on a patient. The suffix may indicate the repair being made or the removal of a body part.

One of the most common surgical suffixes you will encounter is **-ectomy,** meaning the excision or removal of whatever the root word indicates. Think back to our prefix discussion where you learned **ec-** and **ecto-,** meaning outside. An **-ectomy,** therefore, takes something *outside* the body. Let's examine a few medical terms using the suffix **-ectomy:**

**TONSILL/ECTOMY** (ton″sĭ-lek′to-me)—removal of the tonsils

**APPEND/ECTOMY** (ap″en-dek′to-me)—removal of the appendix

**PHLEB/ECTOMY** (fle-bek′to-me)—excision of a vein or a part of a vein

# EXERCISE 1:

In some cases, **-ectomy** may only mean removal of part of an organ or body part because if the entire organ or body part were removed, the patient would suffer. What would the term **hepatectomy** (hep″ah-tek′to-me) indicate to you?

a. removal of a portion of the gallbladder (page 76)
b. removal of a portion of the liver (page 76)

Another suffix you will frequently see is **-(o)tomy**—a surgical incision into whatever body part the root word indicates. Sometimes a patient will be scheduled for an **-(o)tomy** that becomes an **-ectomy** during surgery. For example, an **arthrotomy** (ar-throt′-o-me)—surgical incision of a joint—could become an **arthrectomy** (ar-threk′to-me)—surgical removal of a joint or part of a joint—if the surgeon decided that it would benefit the patient.

# EXERCISE 2:

If we tell you that the stem **cran-** refers to the skull, which term below describes a surgical incision into the skull?

   a.  craniotomy (kran″ne-ot′o-me) (page 76)
   b.  craniectomy (kran″ne-ek′to-me) (page 76)

Other examples using the suffix **-(o)tomy** include

**NEUR/OTOMY** (nu-rot′o-me)—the dissection of a nerve

**THORAC/OTOMY** (tho″rah-kot′o-me)—the opening of the chest

**LAPAR/OTOMY** (lap-ah-rot′o-me)—a surgical incision into the abdominal area
    of the body; specifically below the ribs and above the ilium (the hip bone)

The suffix **-lithotomy** means to make an incision specifically to remove stones from a part of the body. You may remember that the stem part **-lith** means stone. **Cholelithotomy** (ko″le-li-thot′o-me) is the surgical procedure for making an incision into the gallbladder to remove stones. The term **lithotomy** can also stand on its own to mean any surgical procedure to remove stones.

# EXERCISE 3:

What does the term **nephrolithotomy** (nef″ro-li-thot′o-me) mean?

   a.  the removal of stones from the liver (page 76)
   b.  the removal of stones from the kidney (page 76)

The suffix used to describe a surgical puncture with a needle or similar instrument is **-centesis.** Like lithotomy, **centesis** can stand on its own or be attached to a root word. Sometimes there will be something withdrawn from the body with the needle, as in the procedure called **amniocentesis** (am″ne-o-sen-te′sis)—the puncture of the uterus to obtain amniotic fluid during pregnancy. Frequently the term **paracentesis** (par″ah-sen-te′sis) will be seen. It refers specifically to the procedure that punctures a *cavity* (for example, the abdominal cavity) to aspirate or withdraw fluid from it.

# EXERCISE 4:

What does **cardiocentesis** (kar″de-o-sen-te′sis) describe?

a. a surgical puncture into the heart (page 77)
b. a surgical removal of part of the heart (page 77)

Other terms that use this suffix are:

**ENTERO/CENTESIS** (en″ter-o-sen-te′sis)—surgical puncture of the intestines

**THORA/CENTESIS** (tho″rah-sen-te′sis)—puncture of the chest wall to withdraw fluid from the pleural cavity

Another surgical procedure involves the insertion of an instrument to look into or examine the inner areas of the body. The suffix used is **-scopy.** The instrument would be a **-scope.** For instance, **cystoscopy** (sis-tos′ko-pe)—looking into the bladder—would be performed by a **cystoscope.** A **bronchoscopy** (brong-kos′ko-pe), which examines the bronchi, however, is done with an **endoscope** (en′do-skōp).

## EXERCISE 5:

Thinking back to what you learned about prefixes, what is an **endoscope?**

a. an instrument that looks into the inside of the intestines (page 77)
b. an instrument that examines the interior of the body (page 77)

## BONUS BRAIN TEASER:

What does a **laparoscopy** (lap″ah-ros′ko-pe) describe?

(Answer on page 77)

Several suffixes are used to describe procedures used in the repair or fixing of the body. Study the suffixes below and the examples:

| SUFFIX | MEANING | EXAMPLE |
|--------|---------|---------|
| **-desis** | binding, fixation | **ARTHRODESIS** (ar″thro-de′sis)—surgical fixation of a joint |
| **-pexy** | suspension, fixation | **HYSTEROPEXY** (his′ter-o-pek-se)—fixation or suspension of the uterus |
| **-plasty** | surgical correction, plastic repair | **ARTHROPLASTY** (ar′thro-plas″te)— reconstruction of a joint |

Let's take a moment to differentiate among these terms. You will see the suffix **-desis** mostly attached to roots that are part of the skeletal–muscular system. It will refer to the fixing or re-affixing of bones, muscles, or joints. **-Pexy,** on the other hand, will be used more with the organs of the body. It describes the procedure used to put the organ back in its original position. The suffix **-plasty** means to redo or perform plastic surgery on a body part. That may sometimes mean adding an artificial part to reform the original shape.

## EXERCISE 6:

Define the following terms:

spondylodesis (spon"dĭ-lod'ĕ-sis) _____ of the spine
hepatopexy (hep"ah-to-pek"se) _____
rhinoplasty (ri'no-plas"te) _____ of the nose
hernioplasty (her'ne-o-plas"te) _____
gastropexy (gas'tro-pek"se) _____

(Answers on page 77)

The suffix **-rhaphy** means joining in a seam or suture. More often you will see a double **r** with this suffix, between the stem and the suffix. Examples of this suffix include:

**PERINEORRHAPHY** (per"ĭ-ne-or'ah-fe)—suture of a perineum (pelvic floor)

**HERNIORRHAPHY** (her"ne-or'ah-fe)—suture of a hernia

## EXERCISE 7:

What does **arteriorrhaphy** (ar'te"re-or'ah-fe) mean?

_____

(Answer on page 78)

To create an artificial opening or mouth, the surgical procedure will be defined by the suffix **-(o)stomy**. The opening that is created is called a **stoma,** which is more or less a permanent opening. A common operation is a **colostomy** (ko-los'to-me) in which an artificial opening is made into the colon and a stoma is created. A colostomy bag is attached to the stoma to collect body wastes. A **gastroenterostomy** (gas"tro-en-ter-os'to-me) is the creation of an artificial opening between the stomach **(gastr-)** and the intestines **(entero-).**

# EXERCISE 8:

Which term describes the creation of an opening into the urinary bladder?

a. cystotomy (sis-tot'o-me) (page 78)
b. cystostomy (sis-tos'to-me) (page 78)

Other surgical suffixes include:

**-SECT**—to cut

**-TRIPSY**—a crushing or friction

To **dissect** something is to cut it apart or separate it from its original form. The surgical suffix **-tripsy** indicates that something is intentionally crushed, as a calculus (stone) in the bladder **(lithotripsy).**

You will learn more about surgical terms in Chapter 14, Surgical Terms and Tools. Continue with the exercise on page 79 before beginning Unit III.

# CHAPTER 4 ANSWERS

**YOUR ANSWER:   1a.**   removal of a portion of the gallbladder

Incorrect. The stem **hepat** refers to the liver rather than the gallbladder. Return to page 70 and select another answer.

**YOUR ANSWER:   1b.**   removal of a portion of the liver

Correct. **Hepatectomy** means to remove only a portion of the liver. To remove the entire liver without a transplant of a new one would be fatal to the patient. As is the case with many medical terms, you will need to realize that this difference exists. You may need to look up terms in a medical dictionary when you are uncertain whether **-ectomy** means removal of the whole or only a portion of the whole. Return to page 71.

**YOUR ANSWER:   2a.**   craniotomy

Correct. A **craniotomy** refers to any surgical operation on the cranium (skull bones of the head). Return to page 71.

**YOUR ANSWER:   2b.**   craniectomy

You are incorrect. **Craniectomy** is the removal of part of the skull. It does not indicate the surgical incision into the skull. Return to page 71 and continue.

**YOUR ANSWER:   3a.**   the removal of stones from the liver

Incorrect. The stem **hepat** means liver. Return to page 71 and look again at the stem of the word.

**YOUR ANSWER:   3b.**   the removal of stones from the kidneys

Correct. The term **nephrolithotomy** means:

> **NEPHRO-+   -LITHOTOMY   =   NEPHROLITHOTOMY**
> (kidney)   (removal of stone)   (operation to remove a stone or
>                                  stones from the kidney)

Return to page 72.

**YOUR ANSWER:    4a.**    a surgical puncture into the heart

Correct. Look at the term more closely:

**CARDIO-** +        **-CENTESIS**        =  **CARDIOCENTESIS**
(heart)        (surgical puncture) .        (surgical puncture
into the heart)

Return to page 72.

**YOUR ANSWER:    4b.**    a surgical removal of part of the heart

Incorrect but close. The suffix **-centesis** describes the procedure to puncture or tap the heart but not necessarily remove a part of the heart, although fluid from the area may be withdrawn. Return to page 72 and continue with answer 4a.

**YOUR ANSWER:    5a.**    an instrument which looks into the insides of the intestines

Incorrect. **Endo-** refers to the interior or inside of a structure, but nothing is mentioned in the term about the intestines. That instrument would be an **enteroscope** (en′ter-o-skōp″)—**enter-** = intestines. Return to page 73 and select another answer.

**YOUR ANSWER:    5b.**    an instrument that examines the interior of the body

Correct. An **endoscope** is used to look into any hollow cavity of the body, such as the bronchi, the bladder, or the esophagus. Return to page 73.

## BONUS BRAIN TEASER, PAGE 73:

A **laparoscopy** describes *an examination into the abdominal area.*

## EXERCISE 6 ANSWERS:

spondylodesis    *fixation (fusion) of the spine*
hepatopexy    *replacement of a "floating" or misplaced liver*
rhinoplasty    *plastic surgery, repair of the nose*
hernioplasty    *surgical repair of a hernia*
gastropexy    *surgical replacement of the stomach*

**EXERCISE 7 ANSWER:**

Arteriorrhaphy means *suture of an artery*.

**YOUR ANSWER:   8a.**   cystotomy

This is incorrect. A cystotomy is a surgical incision into the bladder, as indicated by the suffix -(o)tomy. Return to page 75 and look closely at the suffix.

**YOUR ANSWER:   8b.**   cystostomy

Correct. A **cystostomy** is the creation of an artificial opening into the urinary bladder. Return to page 75.

# CHAPTER 4 SUFFIX WORD STUDY LIST

amniocentesis (am″ne-o-sen-te′sis)
appendectomy (ap″en-dek′tə-me)
arteriorrhaphy (ahr-ter″e-or′ə-fe)
arthrectomy (ar-threk′to-me)
arthrodesis (ar″thro-de′sis)
arthroplasty (ar′thro-plas″te)
arthrotomy (ar-throt′-o-me)
cardiocentesis (kar″de-o-sen-te′sis)
centesis (sen-te′sis)
cholelithotomy (ko″le-lĭ-thot′o-me)
colostomy (ko-los′to-me)
cystoscope (sis′to-skōp″)
cystoscopy (sis-tos′ko-pe)
dissect (dĭ-sekt′)
endoscope (en′do-skōp)
enterocentesis (en″tər-o-sənte′sis)
gastroenterostomy (gas″tro-en-ter-os′-
    to-me)
gastropexy (gas′tro-pek″se)
hepatectomy (hep″ah-tek′to-me)

hepatopexy (hep″ah-to-pek″se)
hernioplasty (her′ne-o-plas″te)
herniorrhaphy (her″ne-o-r′ah-fe)
hysteropexy (his′ter-o-pek-se)
laparotomy (lap″ərot′əme)
lithotomy (lĭ-thot′ə-me)
lithotripsy (lith′o-trip″se)
nephrolithotomy (nef″ro-lĭ-thot′-
    o-me)
neurotomy (noō-rot′əme)
paracentesis (par″ah-sen-te′sis)
perineorrhaphy (per″ĭ-ne-or′ah-fe)
phlebectomy (flə-bek′to-me)
rhinoplasty (ri′no-plas″te)
spondylodesis (spon″dĭ-lod′ĕ-sis)
stoma (sto′mə)
thoracentesis (thor″ə-sen-te′sis)
thoracotomy (thor″ə-kot′ə-me)
tonsillectomy (ton″sĭ-lek′tə-me)

## SUFFIX EXERCISE

Define the following terms:

1. gastralgia _____
2. arthralgia _____
3. anemia _____
4. dermatitis _____
5. gastrectomy _____
6. pneumectomy _____
7. neurology _____

8. tracheotomy _____
9. leukemia _____
10. esophagoscopy _____
11. nephropexy _____
12. splenopexy _____
13. neuroplasty _____
14. blepharoplasty _____ of the eyelid
15. cardiology _____
16. dermatology _____
17. arthritis _____
18. suffix _____
19. cholelithiasis _____
20. colostomy _____

Write the medical term which the definition describes:

1. Inflammation of the heart _____
2. Excision or removal of a joint _____
3. Inflammation of the brain—encephal _____
4. Science of the stomach and intestines _____
5. Blood poisoning _____
6. A surgical puncture of the intestines _____
7. Removal of stones from the kidney _____
   (**Hint:** Use the suffix for removal of stones.)
8. A tumor of a muscle _____
9. The suffix that means to create an artificial opening or
   mouth _____
10. Procedure used to look into the bladder _____

(Answers in Appendix, page 260)

# SUFFIX PUZZLE

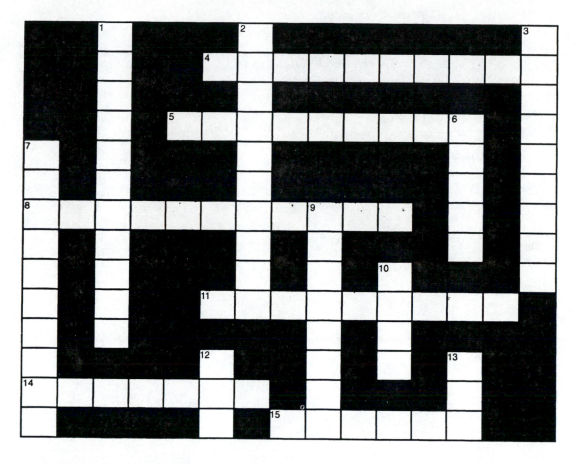

## CLUES FOR SUFFIX PUZZLE

### Across

4. Science and study of the heart
5. Inflammation of an artery
8. Removal of a vein
11. The breaking down of hemoglobin from the red blood cells
14. Suffix for softening
15. Pus in the blood

## Down

1. Surgical repair of the nose
2. Protrusion of the stomach
3. Originating in cells; cell development
6. Suffix for opening or mouth
7. Surgical opening into the abdomen
9. The study of tumors
10. A fluid-filled sac or bladder
12. Suffix for "being like" or resembling
13. Suffix for tumor

(Answers on page 262)

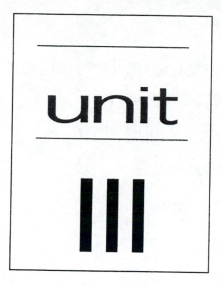

unit

III

# STEMS (ROOT WORDS)

III

# chapter five 5

# Introduction to the Body

## TERM STUDY LIST

adipose

anatomy

cell

connective tissue

edema

epithelial tissue

necrosis

organs

pathology

physiology

system

systemic

tissues

This unit will be an introduction to **stems** (sometimes called root words). We will approach this learning phase through the use of the body **systems.** The unit has been divided into nine chapters for ease in learning the stems associated with each system. Since this is a very basic introductory text, you will learn only the most common stems associated with each system. The text is not meant to be a complete explanation of each system.

A few definitions should be covered before you read further. You will encounter these terms and conditions as you further your study of the human body. The basic part of a living organism is called a **cell.** Many similar cells comprise **tissues,** more complex units. You will find varying and numerous kinds of cells and tissues in your study of the human body. The four basic types of tissues are **epithelial** (ep"ĭ-the'le-al) (covers the body and many of its parts), **connective** (connects parts of the body), **muscle** (provides movement), and **nervous** (special makeup of cells in the brain and nervous system). **Adipose** (ad'ĭ-pōs) or fatty tissue is a type of connective tissue. Some tissues may get an abnormal collection of fluids causing a condition called **edema** (ĕ-de'mah).

Even more complex units are the body's **organs**—a combination of different kinds of tissue. Organs perform the functions of the body. Your heart, liver, stomach, etc. are organs—each has a specific purpose and each is comprised of several kinds of tissue. When several organs work together to perform a specific function of the body, they make up a system. The body systems are the divisions we are using in this unit. A physical problem or disease that is **systemic** affects the whole system of the body. Diagnostic techniques used for identifying changes in tissues and cells are discussed in Chapter 13, beginning on page 201.

To learn even more about the human body, it is suggested that you take an anatomy and physiology course. (Also, a text resource listing on page 278 of this book provides sources for you to consult.) A course in anatomy would teach you the structure of the body and the relationship of the body parts and systems to each other. The physiology part of the course would introduce you to the functions of these parts and what physical and chemical processes take place to make them work. If the body systems and cells are not functioning properly because of disease, the science of **pathology** would be used.

In the study of pathology and diseases, there are numerous terms to be learned. Some of these will be introduced throughout this unit but many will be left for a more in-depth text.

The death of tissue and cells is called **necrosis.** Necrosis can be caused by disease or injury.

# EXERCISE 1:

Break down necrosis and begin using your suffix skills by filling in the blanks.

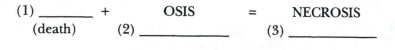

(1) _____ +          OSIS          =          NECROSIS
   (death)          (2) _____          (3) _____

(Answer on page 88)

Development of tissues and cells is not always normal. The term used to describe the lack of development of an organ or tissue is **aplasia.** It could mean an organ is not fully developed or missing altogether. A term to describe the opposite effect of cell growth is **hyperplasia**—the abnormal increase in size of organs or tissues. Again, the prefix makes the difference in term definition!

In this unit you will begin even more word building as you start to reinforce your knowledge of prefixes and suffixes. Before continuing to body systems, you should become familiar with body positioning and anatomical postures. The following sections are identified as 5A, Planes and Direction of Reference; 5B, Terms Describing Direction of Movement; 5-C, Postures; and 5-D, The Human Body Surface Anatomy.

# CHAPTER 5 ANSWERS

**EXERCISE 1:**

     (1) *NEC (R)* +      OSIS      =      NECROSIS

       (death)      (2) (*condition of*)    (3) *cell or tissue death*

# CHAPTER 5 WORD STUDY LIST

adipose (ad'ĭ-pos)
anatomy (ə-nat'ə-me)
aplasia (ə-pla'zhə)
cell (sel)
connective tissue
edema (ə-de'mə)
epithelial (ep"ĭ-the'le-əl) tissue
hyperplasia (hi"pər-pla'zhə)
muscle tissue

necrosis (nə-kro'sis)
nervous tissue
organs (or'gənz)
physiology (fiz"e-ol'ə-je)
stem
system (sis'təm)
systemic (sis-tem'ik)
tissues

# Planes and Direction of Reference

*The planes of the body are often used in the medical field to describe a particular area of the body where disease or injury occurs. Directions of reference are also used in the same manner—to locate a specific area of the body.*

## TERM STUDY LIST

anterior
cauda, caudal
cephalad, cephalic, cephal(o)
distal
dorsal

inferior
lateral
medial, mesial
midline
palmar
peripheral

plantar
posterior
proximal
sagittal
superior
ventral

## Terms Describing Planes and Directions of Reference

For descriptive purposes, the normal anatomical position of the body is **erect,** with the arms hanging by the side and the palms of the hands facing forward, as illustrated in Figure 5A–1.

The first anatomical term describing location that we will deal with is **anterior** (an-te′re-or), which means the ventral, front, or belly surface of the body. It is in contrast to the term **posterior** (pos-te′re-or), which means the dorsal or back surface of the body (see Figure 5A–2).

**Medial** (me′de-al) is the term used to refer to the midline of the body. It is re-

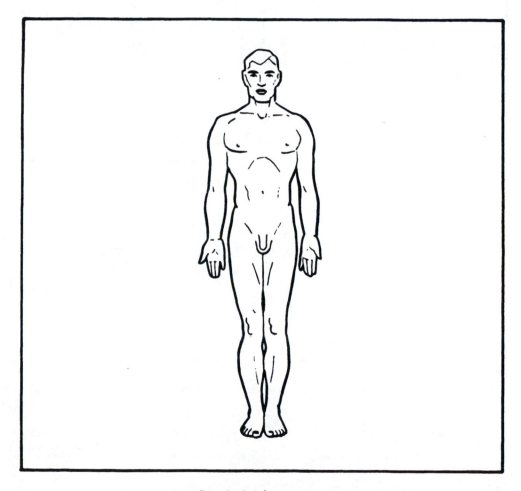

**Figure 5A–1.** Body in erect position

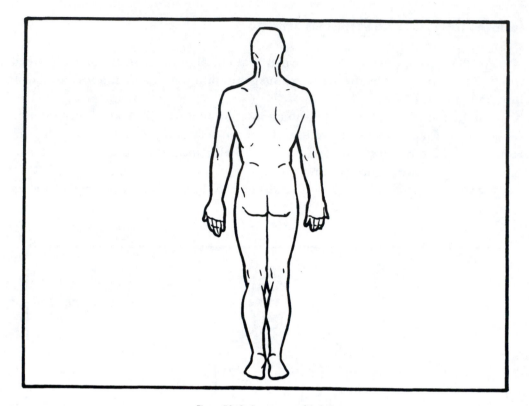

**Figure 5A–2.** Posterior view of the body

lated to the term **sagittal** (saj´ĭ-tal), which is an imaginary plane passing from front through back, dividing the body into right and left portions (see Figure 5A–3).

# EXERCISE 1:

Which view of the human body is shown in Figure 5A–1?

a. anterior (page 99)
b. posterior (page 99)

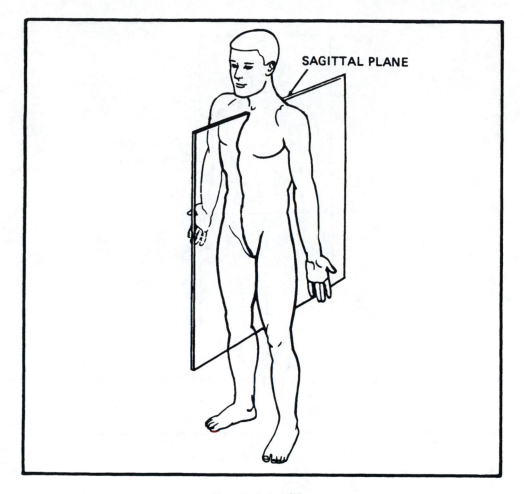

**Figure 5A–3.** Sagittal plane

# EXERCISE 2:

Which medical term means toward the **midline** of the body?

a. lateral (page 99)
b. medial (page 99)

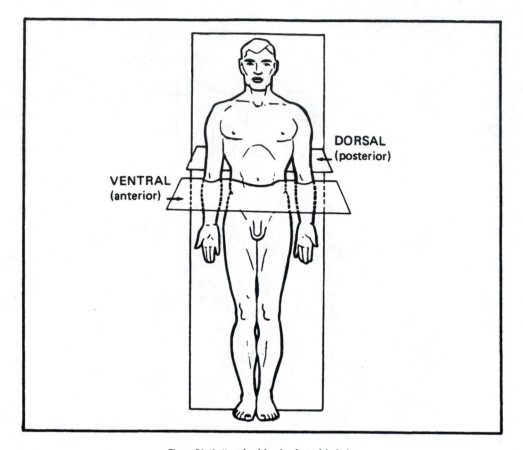

**Figure 5A–4.** Ventral and dorsal surfaces of the body

**Dorsal** (dor'sal) is the term that denotes the back side of the body. The opposite side—or belly side—is called **ventral** (ven'tral). In general, these terms are used interchangeably with the previously discussed terms anterior (ventral—belly side) and posterior (dorsal—back side). The relationship is illustrated in Figure 5A–4.

# EXERCISE 3:

On which surface of the body is the navel located?

a. dorsal (page 99)
b. ventral (page 99)

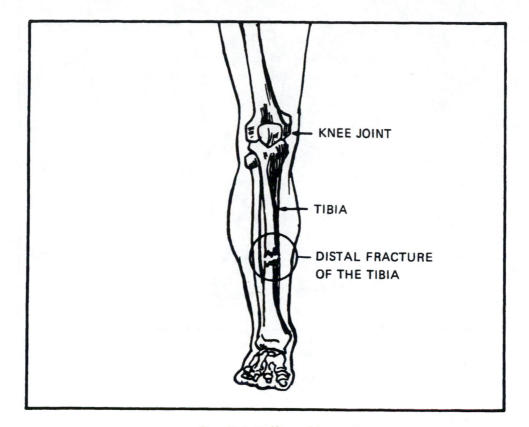

KNEE JOINT

TIBIA

DISTAL FRACTURE
OF THE TIBIA

**Figure 5A–5.** Distal fracture of tibia

Other common terms referring to location are **proximal** (prok′sĭ-mal) (which means nearest the point of origin or attachment) and **distal** (dis′tal) (which means away from the point of origin or attachment). The terms are useful in describing such things as fractures of the limbs as, for example, a fracture occurring at the distal third of the tibia. This means a fracture of the tibia occurring about two-thirds down, below where the tibia is attached to the rest of the leg at the knee (see Figure 5A–5). A proximal fracture would be closer to the point of attachment, the knee in Figure 5A–5. The femur, the large bone of the thigh, is attached to the hip joint (see Figure 5A–6).

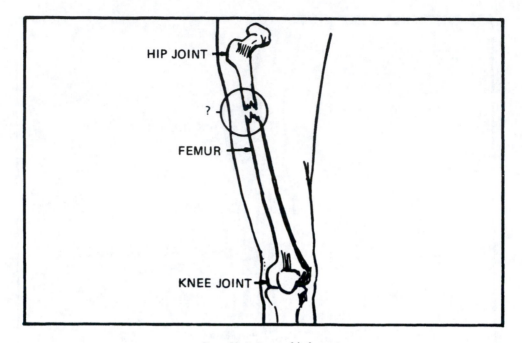

**Figure 5A–6.** Fracture of the femur

# EXERCISE 4:

How would the fracture of the femur shown in Figure 5A–6 be described?

a. fracture of the distal third of the femur (page 100)
b. fracture of the proximal third of the femur (page 100)

You will perhaps have occasion to use the term **peripheral** (pe-rif′er-al). This means at or toward the surface of the body as, for example, the peripheral blood vessels.

Other frequently used terms denoting location are **superior** (su-pe′re-or) (which means toward the head) and **inferior** (in-fe′re-or) (which means toward the feet). You may also encounter the terms **cephalad** (sef′ah-lad), **cephalic**, or **cephalo** which, in addition to superior, refers to the head end of the body; and **cauda**

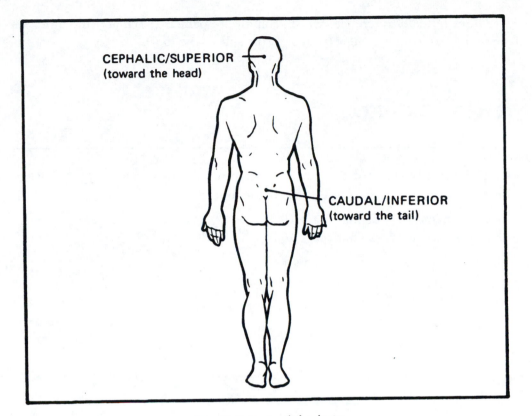

**Figure 5A–7.** Superior and inferior locations

(kaw'dah) or **caudal** (kaw'dal) which, in addition to inferior, refers to locations toward the tail. These directions are illustrated in Figure 5A–7.

# EXERCISE 5:

Given the above information, what do you suppose the term **cephalocaudal** (sef"ah-lo-kaw'dal) means?

    a. Cephalocaudal refers to the bony process extending from the skull to the coccyx (caudal end of the vertebrae). (page 100)

    b. Cephalocaudal refers to the long axis of the body, in a direction from head to tail. (page 100)

Other terms of reference you will employ are **palmar** (pal′mar) (the inner surface of the hand) and **plantar** (plan′tar) (the sole of the foot).

# EXERCISE 6:

The inner surface of the hand is referred to as the (1) _____ surface, whereas (2) _____ refers to the sole of the foot.

a.  (1) palmar (2) plantar (page 100)
b.  (1) plantar (2) palmar (page 100)

# CHAPTER 5A ANSWERS

**YOUR ANSWER:  1a.**   anterior

You are correct. The view shown is one of the anterior, or front surface, of the body.

**YOUR ANSWER:  1b.**   posterior

You are incorrect. The view shown is not a posterior view of the body, since the individual depicted in Figure 5A–1 is **facing** you. Please return to page 92 and select the correct answer from the alternatives provided.

**YOUR ANSWER:  2a.**   lateral

You are incorrect. Lateral does not mean toward the midline of the body. It refers to the left or to the right of the midline, as shown in Figure 5B–1. Please return to page 93 and select the correct answer to the question from the alternatives suggested.

**YOUR ANSWER:  2b.**   medial

You are correct. **Medial** is the term which refers to the midline of the body. You may sometimes hear the term **mesial** (me′ze-al) used for the same purpose. Mesial also means located near the **midline** of the body. Just in passing, it might be well to remember that the midline is used as a reference point for other terms denoting location. For example, as shown in Figure 5B–2, the term **lateral** (lat′er-al) means the surface to the right or left of the midline. Return to page 94.

**YOUR ANSWER:  3a.**   dorsal

You are incorrect. Remember, ventral refers to the front or belly surface of the body, and posterior refers to the back or dorsal surface. Please return to page 94 and select the correct answer from the alternatives provided.

**YOUR ANSWER:  3b.**   ventral

You are correct. The navel, or belly button, is located on the ventral or belly surface of the body. Return to page 95.

**YOUR ANSWER:   4a.**    fracture of the distal third of the femur

You are incorrect. If you will remember, we indicated that distal is defined as **away** from the point of origin or attachment. (In this case the point of attachment is at the hip joint.) Look at Figure 5A–6 again. Does it display a fracture more away from than toward the point of attachment? Please select the correct answer on page 96 before you proceed.

**YOUR ANSWER:   4b.**    fracture of the proximal third of the femur

You are correct. Figure 5A–6 does illustrate a fracture of the proximal third of the femur. We use the term **proximal** because the fracture is nearest to the point of origin or attachment (in this case the hip joint). Return to page 96.

**YOUR ANSWER:   5a.**    cephalocaudal refers to the bony process extending from the skull to the coccyx (caudal end of the vertebrae)

You are incorrect. Cephalocaudal is a term that refers to direction—not to a specific bony process. Please return to page 97 and select the correct answer from the alternatives provided.

**YOUR ANSWER:   5b.**    cephalocaudal refers to the long axis of the body, in a direction from head to tail

You are correct. Cephalocaudal does mean proceeding in a direction from the head toward the tail. Return to page 98.

**YOUR ANSWER:   6a.**    (1) palmar (2) plantar

You are correct. **Palmar** does refer to the inner surface of the hand, and the **plantar** surface of the foot refers to the sole. Continue with Chapter 5B.

**YOUR ANSWER:   6b.**    (1) plantar (2) palmar

You are incorrect. Could it just be possible that you answered without reading the material presented? Please turn back to page 98, read the material again, and select the correct answer from the alternatives provided.

# CHAPTER 5A WORD STUDY LIST

anterior (an-te're-or)
cauda, caudal (kaw'dah), (kaw'dal)
cephalad (sef'ah-lad)
cephalic (sə-fal'ik), cephalo
cephalocaudal (sef"ah-lo-kaw'dal)
distal (dis'tal)
dorsal (dor'sal)
erect (e-rekt')
inferior (in-fe're-or)
medial (me'de-al)

midline
palmar (pal'mar)
peripheral (pe-rif'er-al)
plantar (plan'tar)
posterior (pos-te're-or)
proximal (prok'sĭ-mal)
sagittal (saj'ĭ-tal)
superior (su-pe're-or)
ventral (ven'tral)

# Terms Describing Direction of Movement

*Directions of movement are used to describe how a person can or cannot move parts of the body, especially the limbs. These terms are commonly used by physical therapists and the physicians with whom they work.*

## TERM STUDY LIST

| | | |
|---|---|---|
| abduction | flexion | pronation |
| adduction | lateral rotation | supination |
| extension | medial rotation | |

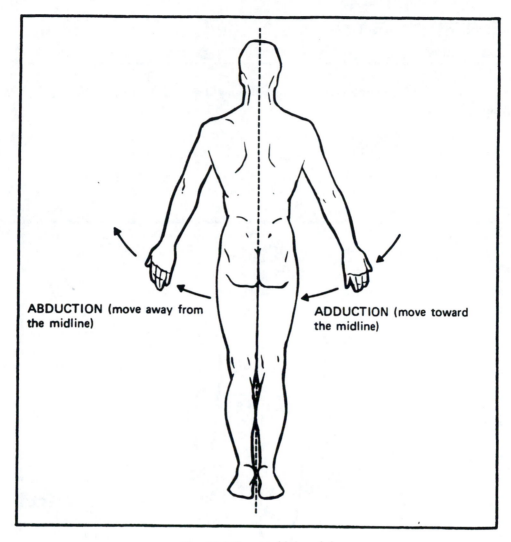

**Figure 5B–1.** Movements of the human body

Abduction (ab-duk'shun) is a descriptive term that indicates movement **away from** the midline. **Adduction** (ah-duk'shun) refers to movement **toward** the midline (see Figure 5B–1).

# EXERCISE 1:

What type of movement would you display if you were to lift your right arm straight out to the side?

a. adduction (page 109)
b. abduction (page 109)

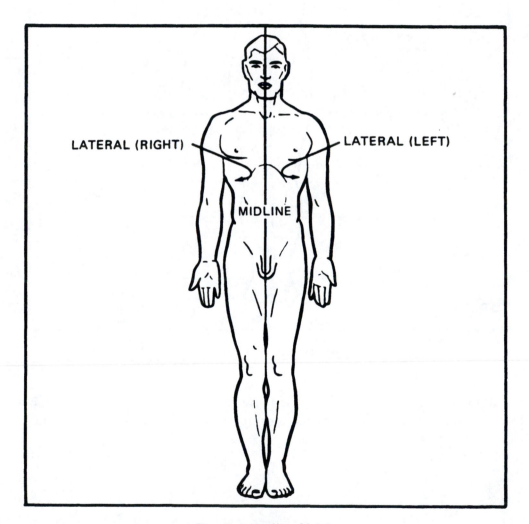

**Figure 5B–2.** Lateral views of the body

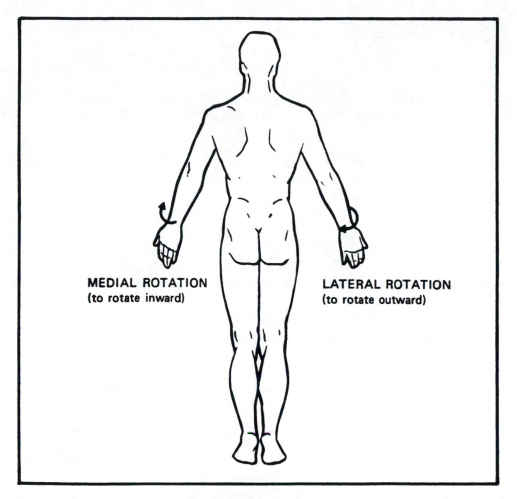

**Figure 5B–3.** Medial and lateral rotation

As previously noted in Chapter 5A, **lateral** means to the side, right or left of the midline (see Figure 5B–2).

**Lateral rotation** means to rotate outward—**away** from the body's midline. **Medial** rotation means to rotate inward—**toward** the body's midline. These movements are illustrated in Figure 5B–3.

# EXERCISE 2:

Stand with your arms at their natural position of rest. Now, rotate your entire right arm so that the palm faces directly to the front. What type of movement did you demonstrate?

a. lateral rotation (page 109)
b. medial rotation (page 109)

**Flexion** (flek'shun) is the term used to describe the act of bending or the condition of being bent. Its opposite term is **extension** (eks-ten'shun), which describes any movement by which the two ends of any part are pulled asunder or which brings the members of an extremity (limb) or the body into or toward a straight condition. Figure 5B–4 illustrates these two conditions.

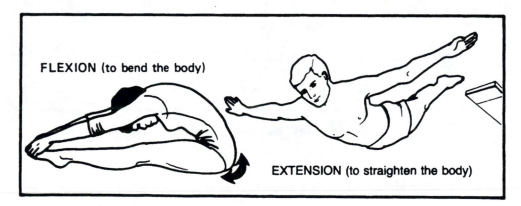

**Figure 5B–4.** Flexion and extension

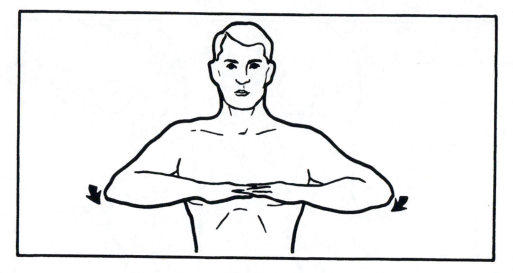

**Figure 5B–5.**

# EXERCISE 3:

Which act (flexion or extension) is illustrated in Figure 5B–5?

a. extension (page 109)
b. flexion (page 109)

In speaking of movements of the forearm and hand, specialized terminology may sometimes be employed. For example, **supination** (su″pi-na′shun) means turning the hand so that the palm faces forward, and **pronation** (pro-na′shun) means turning the palm of the hand backward. These specialized movements are illustrated in Figure 5B–6.

These terms of reference relate to a body standing erect. If you assume a position other than a standing, erect position, visualize yourself as returned to the erect position to classify the movement.

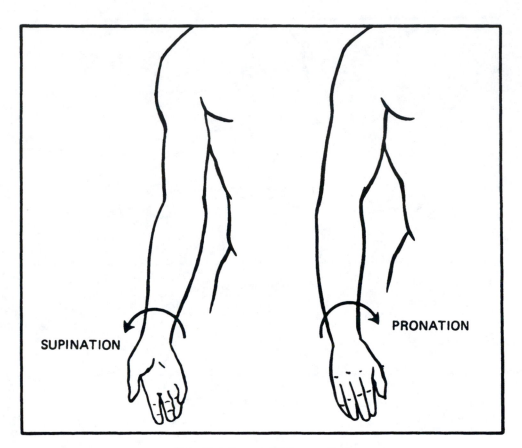

**Figure 5B–6.** Movements of the forearm and hand

## EXERCISE 4:

Place your right hand palm down on your desk or table. Now, rotate it so that the palm faces upward. What type of movement did you demonstrate?

a. supination of the forearm and hand (page 110)
b. pronation of the forearm and hand (page 110)

# CHAPTER 5B ANSWERS

**YOUR ANSWER:  1a.**  adduction

You are incorrect. Adduction describes movement directed toward the midline. Thus, it would define the movement involved in returning the extended arm to its normal resting place at the side of the body. But that's not what the question asked. Please return to page 104 and select the correct answer from the alternatives provided.

**YOUR ANSWER:  1b.**  abduction

You are correct. Abduction does describe the movement involved in lifting the arm straight out to the side. As we stated before, the term literally means to move away from the midline. Return to page 105.

**YOUR ANSWER:  2a.**  lateral rotation

You are correct. The movement you made in rotating your arm is described as lateral rotation—to rotate outward. Return to page 106.

**YOUR ANSWER:  2b.**  medial rotation

You are incorrect. Medial rotation means to rotate inward toward the body's midline—which is just the opposite of the movement you made in rotating your arm. Please return to page 106 and select the correct answer from the alternatives provided.

**YOUR ANSWER:  3a.**  extension

You are incorrect. The position illustrated is NOT one of extension, since the individual in the figure has his arms bent. Please return to page 107 and choose the correct answer from the alternatives provided.

**YOUR ANSWER:  3b.**  flexion

You are correct. The position illustrated is that of flexion—a state in which the arm is bent or flexed. Return to page 107.

**YOUR ANSWER:   4a.**   supination of the forearm and hand

You are correct. The movement you made did illustrate the term supination, which means to turn the hand (and arm) so that its surface is facing forward. Continue with Chapter 5C.

**YOUR ANSWER:   4b.**   pronation of the forearm and hand

You are incorrect. The movement you made was NOT pronation. Pronation, if you will remember, means turning the palm of the hand backward. Please return to page 108, review a bit, and then select the correct answer from the alternatives provided.

# CHAPTER 5B WORD STUDY LIST

abduction (ab-duk'shun)
adduction (ah-duk'shun)
extension (eks-ten'shun)
flexion (flek'shun)

lateral (lat'ər-əl) rotation
medial (me'de-əl) rotation
pronation (pro-na'shun)
supination (su"pi-na'shun)

# chapter five c

# Postures

*There are several positions the body may be placed in for surgical, diagnostic, or therapeutic reasons. These positions yield the terms you will learn in this chapter.*

## TERM STUDY LIST

| | |
|---|---|
| erect | prone |
| laterally recumbent | supine |

The anatomical postures of the body are: **erect** (e-rekt'), **supine** (su'pin), **prone** (prōn), and **laterally recumbent** (lat'er-al-le re-kum'bent).

The **erect** posture is that of the normal body in a standing position. The **supine** posture is the **recumbent** position of the body lying flat on the back, and **prone** lying face down and flat. You see, supine and prone apply equally to the position of the whole body, or of the forearm and hand.

## EXERCISE 1:

Which anatomical posture is illustrated in Figure 5C–1?

a. prone (page 115)
b. supine (page 115)
c. erect (page 115)

Other anatomical postures include the **laterally recumbent** positions (the horizontal position of the body while lying on either the right or the left side). The positions, left laterally recumbent and prone, are illustrated in Figure 5C–2, A and B.

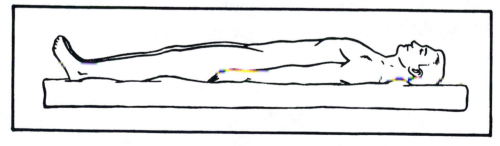

**Figure 5C–1.**

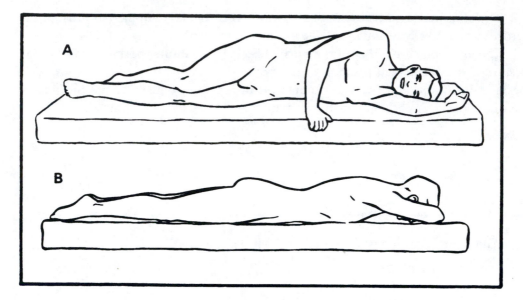

**Figure 5C–2.** Anatomical postures

## EXERCISE 2:

Which positions are shown in Figure 5C–2, A and B?

a. 5C–2A illustrates the supine position; 5C–2B illustrates the prone position (page 115)

b. 5C–2A illustrates the left laterally recumbent position; 5C–2B illustrates the prone position (page 115)

# CHAPTER 5C ANSWERS

---

**YOUR ANSWER:   1a.**   prone

You are incorrect. The posture shown is NOT the prone. The prone position is the horizontal position of the body lying face down—exactly opposite to the posture shown. Please return to page 113 and select the correct answer from the alternatives provided.

**YOUR ANSWER:   1b.**   supine

You are correct. The posture shown is supine—the horizontal position of the body lying flat on its back. Return to page 113.

**YOUR ANSWER:   1c.**   erect

You are incorrect. The erect position is the normal posture of the body in the standing position. The illustration on page 113 certainly doesn't show a person in the erect position! Please return to page 113, and select the correct answer from the alternatives provided.

**YOUR ANSWER:   2a.**   5C–2A illustrates the supine position; 5C-2B illustrates the prone position

You are partly right—5C–2B does illustrate the prone position. However, the position shown in 5C–2A is definitely NOT supine. If you'll remember, we said that the supine position was the horizontal position of the body lying flat on its back. Please return to page 114 and select the correct answer from the alternatives provided.

**YOUR ANSWER:   2b.**   5C–2A illustrates the left laterally recumbent position; 5C–2B illustrates the prone position

You are correct in both instances. In subsequent work you will be introduced to special positions such as Sims' position (or semi-prone position) in which the patient is on the left side and chest, the right knee and leg drawn up, and the left arm along the back (see Figure 5C–3), and Fowler's position (see Figure 5C–4), in which the patient's trunk is raised to form an angle of from 60° to 70° with the horizontal; the knee area is raised to prevent slipping of patient. Continue with Chapter 5D.

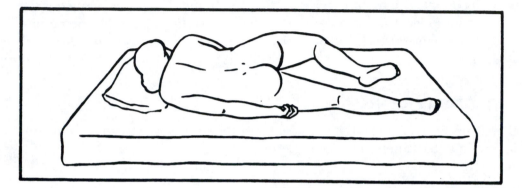

**Figure 5C–3.** Sims' position

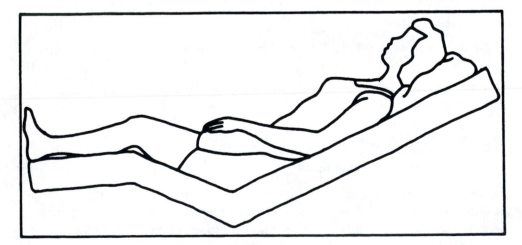

**Figure 5C–4.** Semi-Fowler's position

# CHAPTER 5C WORD STUDY LIST

erect (e-rekt')
laterally recumbent (lat'er-al-le re-
    kum'bent)

prone (prōn)
supine (su'pīn)

# chapter five d

# The Human Body Surface Anatomy

*Shown in Figures 5D–1 and 5D–2 are regions of the body that may be described on a patient's chart or in your further study of the human body. These diagrams are provided for your information. You should already be familiar with most of the terms shown.*

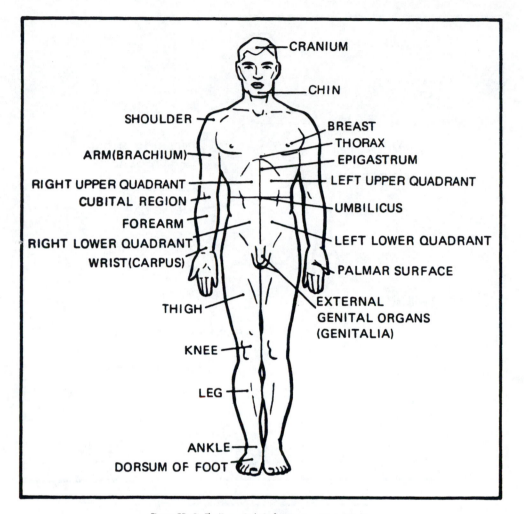

**Figure 5D–1.** The Human Body Surface Anatomy (Ventral View)

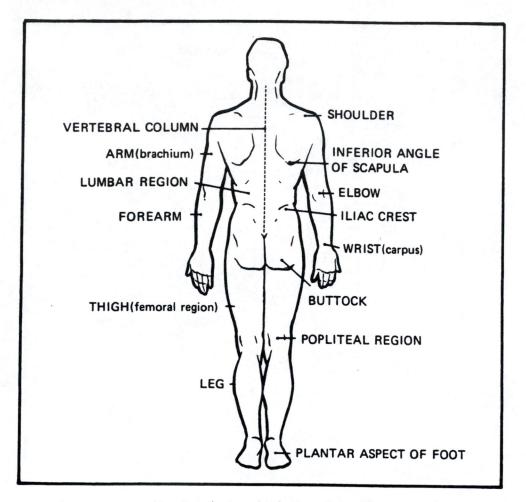

**Figure 5D–2.** The Human Body Surface Anatomy (Dorsal View)

# CHAPTER 5 EXERCISES

## Anatomical Postures

Identify the anatomical postures shown below. Answers on page 264.

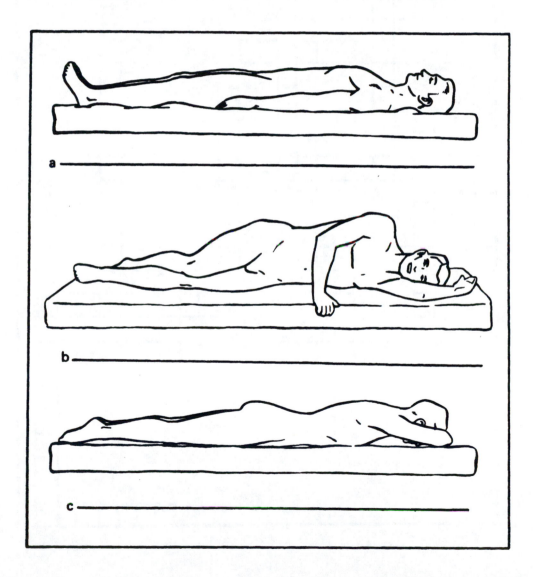

a _____

b _____

c _____

The following pages contain exercises to reinforce your learning of body locations and postures. Try doing as much as you can without referring to the text material. Answers will be found in the Appendix beginning on page 255.

## Crossword Puzzle #1 Body Locations and Positions

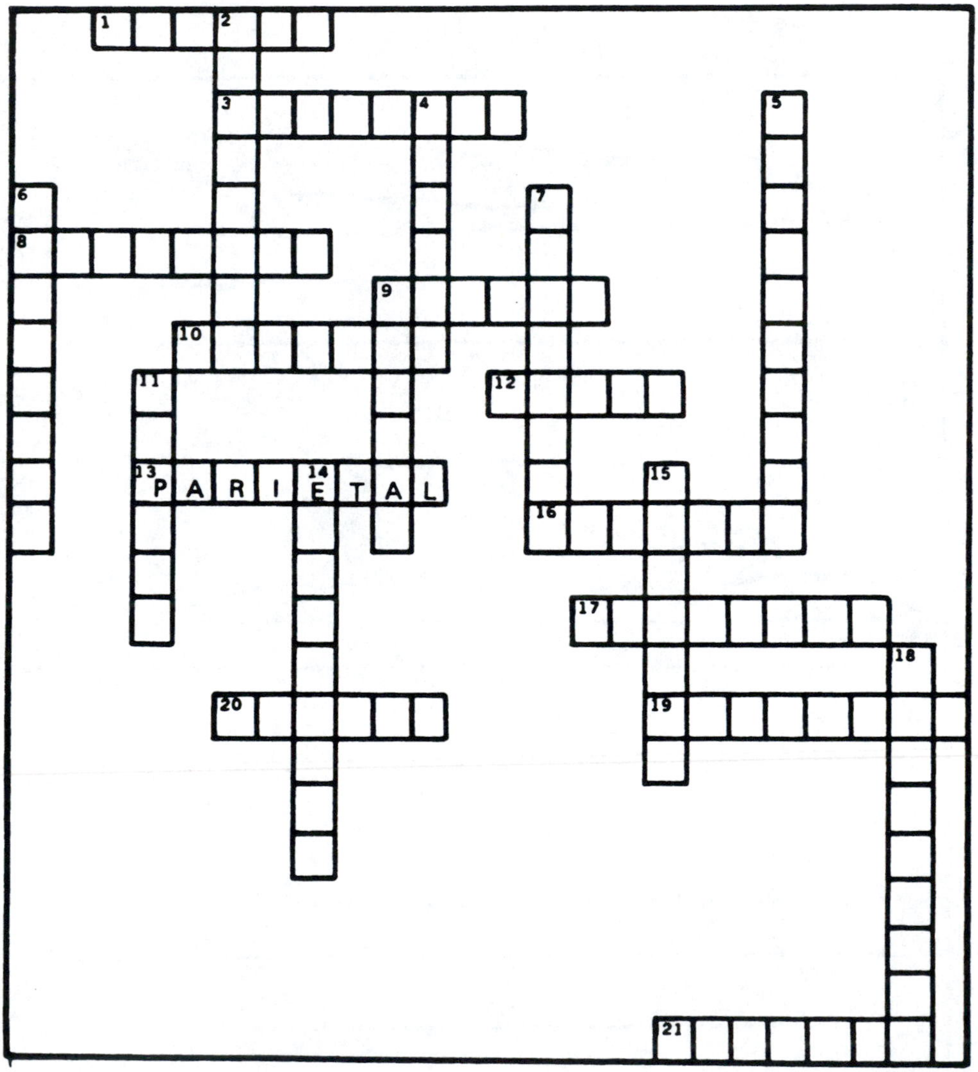

(crossword grid with answer at 13 Across / 13 Down: P A R I E T A L)

# CLUES FOR CROSSWORD PUZZLE—BODY LOCATIONS AND POSITIONS

## Across

1. At or near the back surface of the body or its parts
3. That part that is nearest the point of attachment
8. Beneath or below some part of a surface
9. A hollow place or space in a structure
10. Pertaining to the head or skull
12. Lying face down and flat
13. Pertains to the wall of a structure or a cavity (bonus starter: answer given to you)
16. At or near the side surface of the body or its parts
17. The outside or outer part of a structure
19. Another word for the ventral surface
20. Away from the point of origin or attachment
21. The sole of the foot

## Down

2. Over or above some part of a structure
4. At or toward the midline of the body or its parts
5. At or toward the surface of the body or its parts
6. Pertains to the large interior organs, esp. in the abdomen
7. Refers to the inside or inner part of a structure
9. Away from the head portion of a body; another word for dorsal
11. A position in which the body or its parts are lying on their back surfaces
14. To straighten the body
15. At or near the front surface of the body or its parts
18. Another word for dorsal

# chapter six

# The Circulatory System

*As with the previous chapters, you will be presented a stem and word study list at the beginning of each body system discussion. The first system you will be learning is the circulatory system. Study the root words and terms below briefly before continuing.*

## STEM/TERM STUDY LIST

| | | |
|---|---|---|
| angio- | -emia | sinoatrial |
| arteri(o)- | erythrocyte | splen(o)- |
| atrioventricular | hem- | systole |
| atrium | hemato- | vascular |
| cardi- | leukocyte | venous |
| cyt- | lymph | ventricle |
| diastole | phleb- | |

The **circulatory system** includes the heart, the blood vessels, blood, and the spleen.

You have already learned a lot of terms that use the stem **cardi-,** meaning the heart. **Cardiology** is the science and study of the heart; a **cardiologist** is the physician who specializes in the heart and its related diseases or malfunctions. You may also see the term **coronary** used as a descriptive term in your study of the circulatory system (eg, coronary arteries).

The heart is composed of four chambers or cavities that are called **atria** and **ventricles** (refer to Figure 6–1). They are identified by the side (left or right) of the heart on which they are located. Within the walls of these chambers are the special tissues that control the rhythm of the heartbeat. These are referred to as the **sinoatrial (SA) node** (the pacemaker that starts the process), the **atrioventricular (AV) node,** and a bundle of fibers called the AV bundle or **bundle of His.** They work as a group to create the contractions and relaxations of the heart muscle.

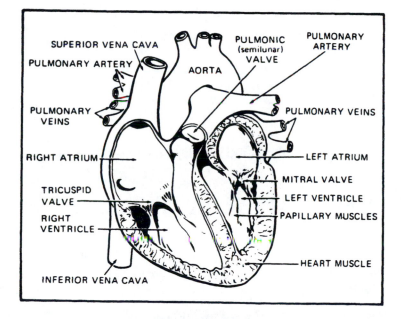

**Figure 6–1.** The heart

# EXERCISE 1:

Areas of the heart that you have learned during your study of prefixes included (1) the **pericardium** and (2) the **endocardium.** Which of the following sets of definitions is correct?

   a. (1) the lining of the heart and (2) the area around the heart (page 133)
   b. (1) the area around the heart and (2) the lining of the heart (page 133)

# EXERCISE 2:

Now write the terms that would mean an inflammation or infection of (1) the pericardium and (2) the endocardium.

   a. _____

   b. _____

(Answers on page 133)

The term that refers to the blood vessels of the body is **vascular.**

# EXERCISE 3:

When added to **cardio-,** what does **cardiovascular** (kar"de-o-vas'ku-lar) describe?

   a. the body's system of arteries, veins, and capillaries (page 133)
   b. the body's system of heart, arteries, veins, and capillaries (page 133)

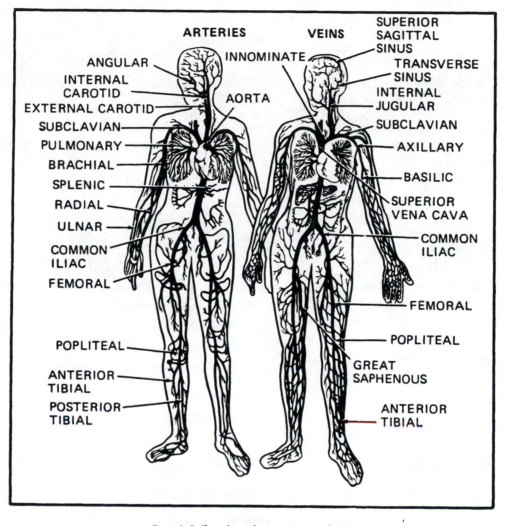

**Figure 6–2.** The cardiovascular system (arteries and veins)

Figure 6–2 shows you this system and identifies important parts of it.

The vascular system includes arteries, veins, and capillaries. The medical stem for arteries is **arteri-.** There are two medical terms that could mean vein: **phleb-** and **venous.** Let's look at a few examples:

**ARTER/ITIS**—inflammation of the arteries

**PHLEB/ITIS**—inflammation of the veins

**INTRA/VENOUS**—within a vein (abbreviated I.V.)

# EXERCISE 4:

What do the terms (1) **arteriectomy** (ar″tĕ-re-ek′to-me) and (2) **phlebectomy** (fle-bek′to-me) indicate to you?

  a. a surgical incision into the (1) arteries and (2) veins (page 134)
  b. the excision or removal of part or all of (1) an artery and (2) a vein (page 134)
  c. the excision or removal of part or all of (1) a vein and (2) an artery (page 134)

Another medical stem that can refer to the vessels is **angio-.** It can refer to the lymph vessels of the body, as well as the blood vessels, but usually means the blood vessels. Examples of common terms include: **angioplasty** (an′je-o-plas″te)—the surgical repair or scraping of blood vessels and **angiogram** (an′je-o-gram″)—an x-ray procedure for looking at the blood vessels.

# EXERCISE 5:

What would the term **angiocarditis** (an″je-o-kar-di′tis) mean?

  a. an inflammation of the blood vessels (page 134)
  b. an inflammation of the heart (page 134)
  c. an inflammation of the heart and blood vessels (page 134)

Now, let's study that red "liquid of life"—blood. There are several terms you have already learned that have used suffixes or stems meaning blood. **Hem-** and **hemat-** are word elements (stems) used to denote blood. No doubt you remember that we also used the stem **-em(ia)** to refer to the blood. **Hematoma** (hem-ah-to′mah) is a medical term meaning a swelling filled with blood, as:

**HEMAT-** +    **-OMA**   =        **HEMATOMA**
(blood)      (swelling)     (swelling containing blood)

Other terms employing the word element include:

**HEMOCYTE** (he'mo-sīt)—a blood corpuscle

**HEMOSTASIS** (he-mos'tah-sis)—checking the flow of blood

**HEMOSTAT** (he'mo-stat)—an instrument for constricting a blood vessel to stop the flow of blood

# EXERCISE 6:

If you are told the stem **gly-** means sugar, what would the following terms mean?

a. hypoglycemia _____

b. hyperglycemia _____

(Answers on page 135)

# EXERCISE 7:

A collection of too much blood in a body part would be:

a. hypoemia (page 135)

b. hyperemia (page 135)

# EXERCISE 8:

What do you think the medical term **hematuria** (hem"ah-tu're-ah) means?

a. blood blister (page 135)

b. blood in urine (page 135)

c. low red blood cell count (page 135)

Blood is made up of plasma, erythrocytes, leukocytes, and thrombocytes. The medical stem **cyt-** refers to cell, making the cell parts of blood easy to learn:

**ERYTHRO/CYTE** (ĕ-rith′ro-sīt)—red blood cell

**LEUKO/CYTE** (look′ko-sīt)—white blood cell

**THROMBO/CYTE** (throm′bo-sīt)—blood platelet (thrombo = clot: platelets aid in clotting)

A cell is the smallest basic unit of living organisms, as we said before. Many different types of cells are found in the human body.

## EXERCISE 9:

What does **cytology** (si-tol′o-je) indicate?

a. the study of blood (page 136)
b. the study of cell life (page 136)

Part of the circulatory system includes the **lymphatic vessels** and **lymph nodes.** In simplest terms, the lymph system is a special part of the circulatory system. It has its own set of capillaries, whose purpose is to wash the tissue cells and provide for body defenses. **Lymphocytes** are nongranular (without grains) leukocytes—also called lymph cells. These lymphocytes are formed in the organ of the body called the spleen.

The medical stem meaning spleen is **splen(o)-.** Let's briefly study a few terms using this stem:

**SPLEN/ECTOMY** (sple-nek′to-me)—removal of the spleen

**SPLENO/MEGALY** (sple″no-meg′ah-le)—enlargement of the spleen

**SPLEN/ITIS** (sple-ni′tis)—inflammation of the spleen

# EXERCISE 10:

_____

What does the term **splenopexy** (sple'no-pek"se) mean?

a.  surgical incision into the spleen (page 136)
b.  surgical fixation of a misplaced spleen (page 136)

A condition that you may encounter in your study of the **cardiovascular (C.V.)** system is an **embolism,** or moving blood clot. It suddenly blocks the flow of blood in an artery. If left there long enough, it can begin to cause death of tissue cells (necrosis) in that area. This is called an **infarction.**

# EXERCISE 11:

_____

Where does a **myocardial infarction (M.I.)** occur? _____

(Answer on page 136)

An **aneurysm** is a sac formed by the dilatation (or bulging) of a wall in an artery, vein, or the heart. It can be caused by an embolism, arteriosclerosis, a physical injury, or infection.

You learned the term arteriosclerosis in your study of suffixes. **Athero-** means the fatty deposits that can build up in arteries.

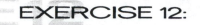

# EXERCISE 12:

Define atherosclerosis. _____

(Answer on page 136)

Two other terms associated with the circulatory system that you will frequently see are **diastole** (di-as′to-le) and **systole** (sis′to-le). The contraction of the ventricles (two of the four chambers of the heart) is called systole; the relaxation phase is called diastole. The two together are measured to give one's blood pressure. The blood pressure reading is written: systolic pressure/diastolic pressure.

# EXERCISE 13:

**Tension** is the pressure applied in this process. By using your prefix knowledge, define the following terms related to the circulatory system:

hypertension _____
hypotension _____
tachycardia _____
bradycardia _____
anemia _____

(Answers on page 136)

Continue with Chapter 7, The Digestive System.

# CHAPTER SIX ANSWERS

**YOUR ANSWER:** **1a.** (1) the lining of the heart and (2) the area around the heart

You are incorrect. You have the two terms reversed. If you remember, the prefix **peri-** means around and the prefix **endo-** means within or inside. Return to page 126 and study the question again.

**YOUR ANSWER:** **1b.** (1) the area around the heart and (2) the lining of the heart

Correct. The pericardium is the area *around* (peri- —around) the heart, and the endocardium is the lining of the heart (endo- —inside, within). Return to page 126.

**EXERCISE 2 ANSWERS:**

  a. inflammation or infection of the pericardium  *pericarditis*
  b. inflammation or infection of the endocardium  *endocarditis*

**YOUR ANSWER:** **3a.** the body's system of arteries, veins, and capillaries

You are incorrect. You picked up only half the term in your answer. Your answer very adequately describes the vascular (vessels) system, but we asked for the *cardiovascular* system. Please return to page 126 and select the correct answer from the alternatives listed.

**YOUR ANSWER:** **3b.** the body's system of heart, arteries, veins, and capillaries

You are correct. The word element **cardio-** does denote heart, and the stem **vascular** does denote the blood vessels. When you put them together into one term you have **cardiovascular,** a very descriptive term for the complicated network of blood vessels and its pump—the heart. Return to page 127.

**YOUR ANSWER: 4a.** a surgical incision into the (1) arteries and (2) veins

You are incorrect. The suffix that indicates a surgical incision is **-otomy.** The suffix we have used here is **-ectomy.** Return to page 128 and select another answer from the alternatives listed.

**YOUR ANSWER: 4b.** the excision or removal of part or all of (1) an artery and (2) a vein

Correct. The suffix **-ectomy** means the excision or removal of all or part of something and in this case means an artery (*arteri*/ectomy) and a vein (*phleb*/ectomy). Return to page 128.

**YOUR ANSWER: 4c.** the excision or removal of part or all of (1) a vein and (2) an artery

You are incorrect. You have the suffix correct but the stems confused. Look at the terms on page 127 again and select another answer.

**YOUR ANSWER: 5a.** an inflammation of the blood vessels

Incorrect. **Angio-** does refer to the blood vessels but the stem **cardi-** (heart) is in the word also. Return to page 128 and select a different answer.

**YOUR ANSWER: 5b.** an inflammation of the heart

This is incorrect. The stem **cardi-** is in the term, meaning heart, but you also have another stem to consider. Return to page 128 and continue.

**YOUR ANSWER: 5c.** an inflammation of the heart and blood vessels

Correct. This is a medical term with two stems:

| **ANGIO-** + | **CARD-** + | **-ITIS** | = | **ANGIOCARDITIS** |
|:---:|:---:|:---:|:---:|:---:|
| (vessels) | (heart) | (inflammation of) | | (inflammation of the blood vessels and heart) |

Return to page 128.

## EXERCISE 6:

a. hypoglycemia   *too little sugar in the blood*
b. hyperglycemia   *too much sugar in the blood*

**YOUR ANSWER:   7a.**   hypoemia

You are incorrect. Remember the prefix **hypo-** means too low or too little? The correct answer is listed below. Read it and return to page 129.

**YOUR ANSWER:   7b.**   hyperemia

You are correct. The prefix **hyper-** means too much or elevated; therefore, hyperemia means too much blood collected in a body part. Return to page 129.

**YOUR ANSWER:   8a.**   blood blister

You are incorrect. The medical term **hematoma** would more accurately describe the condition of a blood blister, since it means a swelling filled with blood. We mentioned the stem **ur(ia)** in an earlier chapter (albuminuria). Does it ring a bell? Please return to page 129 and select the correct answer from the alternatives listed.

**YOUR ANSWER:   8b.**   blood in urine

You are correct. Hematuria does mean blood in the urine, as:

**HEMAT- + -UR(IA)  =  HEMATURIA**
(blood)    (urine)    (blood in urine)

Return to page 130.

**YOUR ANSWER:   8c.**   low red blood count

You are incorrect. The medical term describing low red blood cell count is **anemia** (or an + -emia), which literally means without blood. This may be a deficiency in the total amount of red blood cells, a deficiency in the quantity of blood itself, a deficiency in the quantity or quality of hemoglobin, or inherent defects in the blood cells. Needless to say, anemia is not the condition we're interested in at the moment. You should be able to select the correct answer, since you know that **hemat(o)-** refers to blood and we used **-uria** in a previous exercise. Please return to page 129 and try again.

**YOUR ANSWER: 9a.** the study of blood

You are incorrect. Although there are blood cells, there are also many other types of cells that may be studied; thus, cytology is not limited to the study of blood cells alone. Continue on page 130.

**YOUR ANSWER: 9b.** the study of cell life

You are correct. **Cytology** is the study or science of cell life. All types of cells may be included in the study. Return to page 130.

**YOUR ANSWER: 10a.** surgical incision into the spleen

You are incorrect. The suffix **-otomy** means incision, so the term this phrase describes is a **splenotomy.** Return to page 131 and select the correct answer from the choices listed.

**YOUR ANSWER: 10b.** surgical fixation of a misplaced spleen

Correct. A splenopexy would be the surgical reaffixing of the spleen that was not in its proper place. Return to page 131.

**EXERCISE 11 ANSWER:** *A myocardial infarction occurs in the heart muscle.*

**EXERCISE 12 ANSWER:**

atherosclerosis *fatty deposits (plaque) collect and harden in the arteries*

**EXERCISE 13 ANSWERS:**

hypertension *abnormally high blood pressure*
hypotension *abnormally low blood pressure*
tachycardia *rapid heartbeat*
bradycardia *slow heartbeat*
anemia *low number of erythrocytes (red blood cells)*

# CHAPTER SIX CIRCULATORY SYSTEM STUDY LIST

anemia (ə-ne′me-ə)

aneurysm (an′u-ruzm)

angiocarditis (an″je-o-kar-di′tis)

angiogram (an′je-o-gram″)

angiography (an″je-og′rə-fe)

angioplasty (an′je-o-plas″te)

arteriectomy (ar″tĕ-re-ek′to-me)

arteritis (ahr″tə-ri′tis)

atherosclerosis (ath″ər-o-sklə-ro′sis)

atrioventricular (AV) (a″tre-o-ven-trik′u-lər) node

atrium (a′tre-əm)

bradycardia (brad″e-kar′de-ah)

bundle of His

cardiologist (kahr″de-ol′ə-jist)

cardiology (kahr″de-ol′ə-je),

cardiovascular (C.V.) (kar″de-o-vas′ku-lar)

coronary (kor′ə-nar″e)

cytology (si-tol′o-je)

diastole (di-as′to-le)

embolism (em′bə-liz-əm)

endocardium (en″do-kahr′de-um)

endocarditis (en″do-kahr-di′tis)

erythrocyte (ə-rith′ro-sīt)

hematoma (hem-ah-to′mah)

hematuria (hem″ah-tu′re-ah)

hemocyte (he′mo-sīt)

hemostasis (he-mos′tah-sis)

hemostat (he′mo-stat)

hyperemia (hi″pər-e′me-ə)

hyperglycemia (hi″pər-gli-se′me-ə)

hypertension (hi″pər-ten′shən)

infarction (in-fahrk′shən)

intravenous (I.V.) (in″trə-ve′nəs)

leukocyte (loo′ko-sīt)

lymphatic (lim-fat′ik) vessels

lymph (limf) nodes

lymphocytes (lim′fo-sītz)

myocardial infarction (M.I.) (mi″-o-kahr′dəe-əl in-fahrk′shən)

pericarditis (per″ĭ-kar-di′tis)

pericardium (per″ĭ-kar′de-um)

phlebectomy (fle-bek′to-me)

phlebitis (flə-bi′tis)

sinoatrial (si″no-a′tre-əl) (SA) node

splenectomy (sple-nek′ə-me)

splenitis (sple-ni′tis)

splenomegaly (sple″no-meg′ə-le)

splenopexy (sple′no-pek″se)

systole (sis′to-le)

tachycardia (tak″e-kar′de-ah)

tension (ten′shən)

thrombocyte (throm′bo-sīt)

vascular (vas′ku-lər)

venous (ve′nəs)

ventricle (ven′tri-kəl)

# chapter seven

# 7

# The Digestive System

*This chapter introduces the digestive system—the system that processes the food and drink we intake. We will follow the process starting from the mouth.*

## STEM/TERM STUDY LIST

| | | |
|---|---|---|
| ante cibum | enter- | lip- |
| chole- | gastr- | phag(o)- |
| colo- | glyco- | post cibum |
| dent(o)-, odonto- | hepat- | stalsis |
| emesis | ileum, ileo- | viscer- |

The **digestive system** of the body includes all the parts involved in digestion, from the mouth to the intestines. The stem that is used to mean eat is **phag(o)-**. A person who does not eat is **aphagic** (ah-fa'jik). This may sometimes be a refusal to eat or inability to eat. One of the first places that digestion starts is with the mouth and teeth. The medical stems for anything relating to the teeth are **dent(o)-** and **odont(o)-**. You already know that a dentist is a degreed specialist dealing with the teeth.

# EXERCISE 1:

A dentist uses an **odontoscope.** Which of the following best fits the description of an odontoscope?

    a. an instrument that drills into the teeth (page 144)

    b. an instrument that helps to examine the teeth and mouth (page 144)

After leaving the mouth, the food travels down the **esophagus** (meaning to carry food) to the stomach. You have seen several words with the stem **gastr-** already. **Gastr-** is used in words relating to the stomach.

# EXERCISE 2:

See if you can define the following terms:

1. gastritis _____
2. gastrectomy _____
3. gastrostomy _____
4. gastroscope _____

(Answers on page 144)

From the stomach the food enters the small intestines. It is moved along the intestines by a process called **peristalsis**—a wave-like contraction. During this journey, **metabolism** occurs. Metabolism is the combination of many chemical reactions necessary to use the food to keep the body living. These reactions occur in cells throughout the body, not only in the digestive system, but many of them take place in the intestines. The stem used to refer to the intestines (both large and small) is **enter-**. An example is **enteritis** (en"ter-i'tis)—inflammation of the intestines. A part of the small intestines that we mentioned much earlier in the text is the **ileum** or the terminal portion of the small intestine. The stem used to refer to this section is **ile-**. Another part of the lower intestines is the colon (or large intestines), which appears as **col(o)-** in medical terminology. An artificial opening into the colon is called a **colostomy**. Some procedures are combinations of the different parts of the intestinal tract.

# EXERCISE 3:

Define these terms:

1. ileostomy (il"e-os'to-me) _____
2. gastroenterology (gas"tro-en"ter-ol'o-je) _____
3. enterocolitis (en"ter-o-ko-li'tis) _____
4. colonoscope (ko-lon'o-skōp) _____
5. enterectomy (en"ter-ek'to-me) _____

(Answers on page 144)

One exception to the use of the stem **enter-** is in the term **gastrointestinal (G.I.),** pertaining to the stomach and intestines.

As food moves through the small intestines, digestive juices are added to it, as well as pancreatic fluid and bile (a fluid from the liver). The pancreas, liver, and gallbladder are important at this point in digestion. The pancreas and terms relating to it still use pancreas—it has no special medical stem. The liver and the gallbladder do, however. Terms referring to the liver use **hepat-,** a stem you have seen previously. Terms that refer to the bile secreted by the liver and stored in the gallbladder use the stem **chole-**. Another term for gallbladder is **cholecyst** (ko'le-sist):

$$\underset{\text{(bile, gall)}}{\textbf{CHOLE-}} + \underset{\text{(fluid-filled sac)}}{\textbf{-CYST}} = \underset{\text{(gallbladder)}}{\textbf{CHOLECYST}}$$

# EXERCISE 4:

---

Which of the following definitions fit the words (1) hepatitis (hep"ah-ti'tis) and (2) cholecystitis (ko"le-sis-ti'tis)?

    a. inflammation of the (1) liver and (2) gallbladder (page 144)

    b. inflammation of the (1) gallbladder and (2) the liver (page145)

After leaving the small intestines, the food has dispersed all of its beneficial proteins, amino acids, sugars, fats, etc., and all that is left are waste products, which enter the large intestines. After going through the large intestines, the wastes leave the body through the rectum or the kidneys, for which you will learn the terms in Chapter 8 in the section on the genitourinary system.

If the digestive system is not working properly, it could cause **emesis,** or vomiting.

# EXERCISE 5:

---

What does the term **hyperemesis** (hi"per-em'e-sis) mean?

    a. little or no vomiting (page 145)

    b. excessive vomiting (page 145)

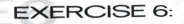EXERCISE 6:

Now, try your luck on the following terms:

1. pericholecystitis (per″ĭ-ko″le-sis-ti′tis) _____

2. cholelithiasis (ko″le-lĭ-thi′ah-sis) _____

3. hepatectomy (hep″ah-tek′to-me) _____

4. hepatopexy (hep′ah-to-pek″se) _____

5. cholecystectomy (ko″le-sis-tek′to-me) _____

(Answers on page 145)

Two other stems that you may see in relation to the digestive system are **glyco-,** meaning sugar or sweet, and **lip-,** referring to fats. **Hypoglycemia** (hi″po-gli-se′-me-ah) means too little blood sugar. **Lipoma** (lĭ-po′mah) is a tumor composed of fat cells.

The terms **ante cibum (a.c.)** and **post cibum (p.c.)** are frequently seen when discussing a patient's meals. The term **a.c.** means before meals (**ante-,** before), and **p.c.** means after meals (**post-,** after)—used mostly in reference to when a medication should be taken.

Although not necessarily related to the digestive system, this is a good time to introduce the stem **viscer(o)-** to you. **Viscero-** means relating to any organs of the body. The digestive system is a part of the **abdominal viscera,** the organs contained in the abdominal cavity. The term **visceral** pertains to *any* internal organ.

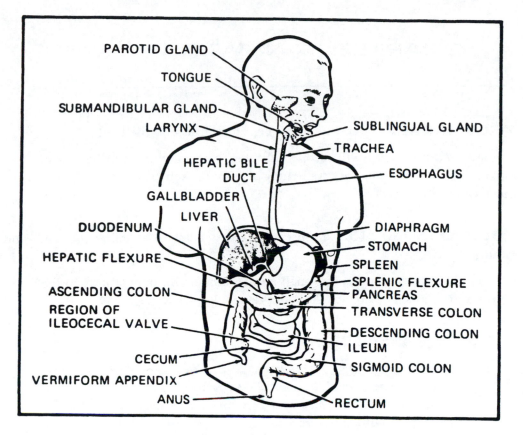

**Figure 7–1.** The digestive system

# BONUS BRAIN TEASER:

Break down this term to identify its meaning: **esophagogastroduodenoscopy** (ǝ-sof″ǝ-go-gas″tro-doo″od-ǝ-nos′kǝ-pe) **(EGD)** (**Hint:** Figure 7–1 may be useful.) _____

(Answer on page 145)

Continue with Chapter 8, Internal Systems.

# CHAPTER 7 ANSWERS

**YOUR ANSWER:** **1a.** an instrument that drills into the teeth

You are incorrect. The suffix **-scope** indicates that something will be examined or looked into, if you remember your study of suffixes. Return to page 139 and select the correct answer.

**YOUR ANSWER:** **1b.** an instrument that helps to examine the teeth and mouth

Correct. An **odontoscope** is the small mouth mirror the dentist uses to look into your mouth. The clue here was the suffix **-scope.** Return to page 139.

## EXERCISE 2 ANSWERS:

1. gastritis   *inflammation of the stomach*
2. gastrectomy   *removal of all or part of the stomach*
3. gastrostomy   *creation of an artificial opening into the stomach*
4. gastroscope   *instrument used to look into the stomach*

## EXERCISE 3 ANSWERS:

1. ileostomy   *creation of an artificial opening into the ileum region of the small intestines*
2. gastroenterology   *science of the stomach and the intestines*
3. enterocolitis   *inflammation of the intestines and the colon*
4. colonoscope   *instrument used to look into the colon*
5. enterectomy   *removal of part of the intestines*

**YOUR ANSWER:** **4a.** inflammation of the (1) liver and (2) gallbladder

Correct. **Hepatitis** is inflammation of the liver and cholecystitis is an inflammation of the gallbladder. Return to page 141.

**YOUR ANSWER:   4b.**   inflammation of the (1) gallbladder and (2) the liver

You are incorrect. You have the two stems confused. Review the material on page 141 again and answer the question again.

**YOUR ANSWER:   5a.**   little or no vomiting

You are incorrect. Remember that the prefix **hyper-** means excessive or too much, and **hypo-** means too little. Return to page 141 and select another answer.

**YOUR ANSWER:   5b.**   excessive vomiting

Correct. The prefix **hyper-** indicates excessive or too much. Hyperemesis, therefore, is excessive vomiting. Return to page 142.

## EXERCISE 6 ANSWERS:

1. pericholecystitis   *inflammation of the area around the gallbladder*
2. cholelithiasis   *condition of gallstones*
3. hepatectomy   *removal of a portion of the liver*
4. hepatopexy   *surgical repair (fixation) of the liver*
5. cholecystectomy   *removal of the gallbladder*

## BONUS BRAIN TEASER:

esophagogastroduodenoscopy   *an internal examination of the esophagus, stomach, and duodenum*

# CHAPTER 7 DIGESTIVE SYSTEM STUDY LIST

abdominal viscera (ab-dom′ĭ-nəl vis′-ər-ə)

ante cibum (a.c.) (an″te si′bəm)

aphagic (ah-fa′jik)

cholecyst (ko′le-sist)

cholecystectomy (ko″le-sis-tek′to-me)

cholelithiasis (ko″le-lĭ-thi′ah-sis)

colonoscope (ko-lon′o-skōp)

colostomy (kə-los′tə-me)

emesis (em′ə-sis)

enterectomy (en″ter-ek′to-me)

enteritis (en″ter-i′tis)

enterocolitis (en″ter-o-ko-li′tis)

esophagogastroduodenoscopy (EGD) (ə-sof″ə-go-gas″tro-doo″od-ə-nos′-kə-pe)

gastrectomy (gas-trek′tə-me)

gastritis (gas-tri′tis)

gastroenterology (gas″tro-en″ter-ol′o-je)

gastrointestinal (G.I.) (gas″tro-in-tes′tĭ-nəl)

gastroscope (gas′tro-skōp)

gastrostomy (gas-tros′tə-me)

hepatectomy (hep″ah-tek′to-me)

hepatopexy (hep′ah-to-pek″se)

hyperemesis (hi″per-em′ĕ-sis)

hypoglycemia (hi″po-gli-se′me-ah)

ileostomy (il″e-os′to-me)

lipoma (lĭ-po′mah)

metabolism (mə-tab′ə-liz″əm)

odontoscope (o″don-to′skōp)

pericholecystitis (per″ĭ-ko″le-sis-ti′tis)

peristalsis (per″ĭ-stal′sis)

post cibum (p.c.) (post si′bəm)

visceral (vis′ər-əl)

# Internal Systems: Endocrine, Genitourinary, and Male/Female Reproductive

*These three systems are being presented as one chapter because their functions are interrelated. Study each system and work the exercises as you go.*

## THE ENDOCRINE SYSTEM

The **endocrine system** provides control and communication for the glands of the body. In this section, you will learn the terms associated with this system.

## STEM/TERM STUDY LIST

| | | |
|---|---|---|
| aden– | exocrine | pituitary |
| adrenal | pancreas | thyroid |
| endocrine | parathryoid | |

The **endocrine** (en'do-krīn) system involves the ductless glands of the body—those glands that secrete their hormones directly into the blood instead of a duct, as the **exocrine** (ek'so-krin) glands do. The two names of the gland systems are good examples of medical terminology:

$$\underset{\text{(within, inside)}}{\text{\textbf{ENDO-}}} \quad + \quad \underset{\text{(secretion)}}{\text{\textbf{-CRINE}}} \quad = \quad \underset{\substack{\text{(hormone is secreted directly} \\ \text{into the bloodstream)}}}{\text{\textbf{ENDOCRINE}}}$$

$$\underset{\text{(outside)}}{\text{\textbf{EXO-}}} \quad + \quad \underset{\text{(secretion)}}{\text{\textbf{-CRINE}}} \quad = \quad \underset{\substack{\text{(hormone is secreted into a duct} \\ \text{to be carried outside the gland)}}}{\text{\textbf{EXOCRINE}}}$$

Study the drawing of the endocrine glands (Figure 8–1) to learn the names and locations of the specific glands. The stem for gland is **aden-. Adenic** (ah-de'nik)

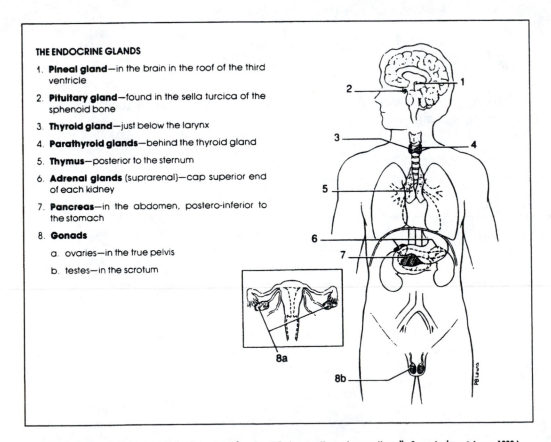

**THE ENDOCRINE GLANDS**

1. **Pineal gland**—in the brain in the roof of the third ventricle

2. **Pituitary gland**—found in the sella turcica of the sphenoid bone

3. **Thyroid gland**—just below the larynx

4. **Parathyroid glands**—behind the thyroid gland

5. **Thymus**—posterior to the sternum

6. **Adrenal glands** (suprarenal)—cap superior end of each kidney

7. **Pancreas**—in the abdomen, postero-inferior to the stomach

8. **Gonads**

   a. ovaries—in the true pelvis

   b. testes—in the scrotum

**Figure 8–1.** The endocrine system. (Used with permission from Guy, J.F., *Learning Human Anatomy*, Norwalk, Conn.: Appleton & Lange, 1992.)

means resembling or pertaining to a gland; **adenitis** (ad"ĕ-ni'tis) is inflammation of a gland; **lymphadenitis** (lim-fad"ĕ-ni'tis) is the inflammation of lymph glands.

# EXERCISE 1:

What should **adenectomy** (ad"ĕ-nek'to-me) signify?

a. surgical removal of the adenoids (page 157)
b. surgical removal of a gland (page 157)
c. surgical removal of an adhesion (page 157)

Some examples of endocrine glands include the **thyroid** and the **parathyroid** (para = behind; located behind the thyroid glands), which are important for body metabolism. The **pituitary gland** helps regulate the thyroid or other endocrine glands that limit or stimulate body growth. You have already learned that the pancreas is important in digestion. The **pancreas** is an endocrine gland.

An endocrine gland that we introduced to you in our discussion of prefixes is the **adrenal gland.**

# EXERCISE 2:

Where is the **adrenal gland** located?

a. in front of the kidneys (page 157)
b. near, on top of the kidneys (page 157)

## THE GENITOURINARY SYSTEM (INCLUDING MALE/FEMALE REPRODUCTIVE TERMS)

Our next system of study is called the **genitourinary** (jen"i-to-u'ri'nar-e) system. This system takes in the male and female reproductive systems and the urinary system that carries off the waste products of digestion.

# STEM/TERM STUDY LIST

| | | |
|---|---|---|
| cysto- | ovum | testes |
| hyster- | perineum | ureter |
| metr- | proct- | urethra |
| nephr- | pyel- | vagina |
| oo- | ren- | vas deferens |
| oophor- | salpingo- | vulva |
| ovaries | | |

Let's look at the **urinary** system first (note Figure 8–2). The most important part of this system is the kidneys. Two different stems may be used to refer to the kidneys: **nephr(o)-** and **ren-**. **Nephralgia** (ne-fral'je-ah) is a pain in the kidneys; **renal** means pertaining to the kidneys.

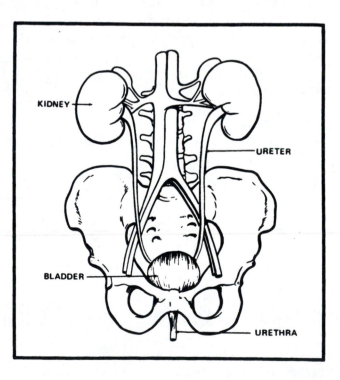

**Figure 8–2.** The urinary system (Modified, with permission, from Cunningham, F.G., MacDonald, P.C., Gant, F.G. *William's Obstetrics* [18th ed.]. Norwalk, Conn.: Appleton & Lange, 1989, p. 85.)

# EXERCISE 3:

Identify the following terms:

1. nephritis (ne-fri′tis) _____
2. nephropexy (nef′ro-pek″se) _____
3. nephroma (ne-fro′ma) _____
4. renointestinal (re″no-in-tes′ti-nal) pertaining to the _____ and _____
5. nephrolithiasis (nef″ro-li-thi′ah-sis) _____

(Answers on page 158)

There is a part of the kidney called the renal pelvis. The medical stem for pelvis is **pyelo-**. **Pyelitis** (pi″ĕ-li′tis) would be an inflammation of the pelvis of the kidney.

# EXERCISE 4:

What would the term **nephropyelolithotomy** (nef″ro-pi″ĕ-lo-lĭ-thot′o-me) mean?

   a. surgical incision for the removal of a stone from the renal pelvis (page 158)
   b. surgical incision into the renal pelvis (page 158)

The stem **cysto-** refers to any fluid-filled bladder or sac but frequently is used to refer to the urinary bladder. **Cystitis** (sis-ti′tis) is an inflammation of the urinary bladder.

# EXERCISE 5:

Define the following terms:

1. cystoscope (sis′to-skōp″) _____
2. nephrocystitis (nef″ro-sis-ti′tis) _____
3. cholecystitis (ko″le-sis-ti′tis) _____

(Answers on page 158)

The tube that connects the kidney with the urinary bladder is the **ureter** (u-re′ter). The **urethra** (u-re′thrah) is the tube which carries urine from the bladder to outside the body. In the male, the end exit is the urethra; in the female, the vulva. The other exit point for body waste products is the **rectum,** or anus. The medical stem for rectum is **procto-.** A **proctoscopy** (prok-tos′ko-pe) is the examination of the rectum using a special instrument called a **proctoscope.** The area between the two exit points is called the **perineum** (per″i-ne′um). When waste products are normally discharged, the process is called **excretion** (note the prefix ex- to mean out— outside the body in this case).

Two medical stems mean **uterus,** an important part of the female reproductive system. They are **metr-** and **hyster-.** The **endometrium** (en-do-me′tre-um) is the membrane lining of the uterus. A **hysterectomy** (his″te-rek′to-me) is the removal of the uterus. The **vagina** is the tube between the uterus and the vulva, as seen in Figure 8–3. **Salpingo-** is the stem that refers to a tube, especially the uterine tube (but also the auditory tube). **Salpingitis** (sal″pin-ji′tis) is an inflammation of the uterine tube through which the eggs travel.

Endocrine glands are also important in reproduction. The **ovaries** and **testes** are endocrine glands. Medical stems for the ovaries and eggs of the female include **oo-, oophor(o)-,** and **ovum.** The element **oo-** and the word **ovum** refer to the female eggs; the stem **oophor(o)-** refers to the ovary itself. An **oophorectomy** is the removal of one or both ovaries, where the eggs are formed.

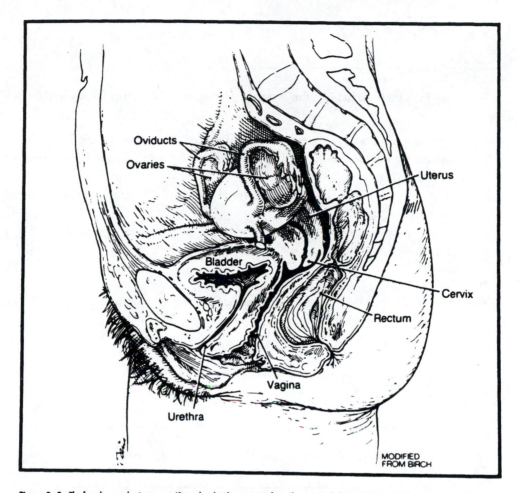

**Figure 8–3.** The female reproductive system (Reproduced with permission from Flynn, J., Hackel, R. *Technological Foundations in Nursing.* Cunningham, F.G., MacDonald, P.C., Gant, F.G., et al. *Williams Obstetrics* [19th ed.]. Norwalk, Conn.: Appleton & Lange, 1993, p. 61.)

## EXERCISE 6:

From what you just learned about these stems, what would a **salpingo-oophorectomy** (sal-ping″go-o″-of-o-rek′to-me) be? _____

(Answer on page 158)

## EXERCISE 7:

What is (1) **metrorrhagia** (me"tro-ra'je-ah) and (2) **hysteropexy** (his'ter-o-pek-se)?

a. (1) uterus pain and (2) surgical replacement of the uterus (page 158)
b. (1) bleeding or excessive flow from the uterus and (2) surgical puncture of the uterus (page 159)
c. (1) bleeding or excessive flow from the uterus and (2) surgical replacement of the uterus (page 159)

The term **natal** relates to birth. The **prenatal** period in a woman's reproductive life is the time when she is pregnant but before she gives birth.

## EXERCISE 8:

By using a variety of prefixes you have already learned, identify the following:

perinatal _____
postnatal _____
neonatal _____ (Hint: neo- = new)

(Answers on page 159)

In the male reproductive system, the **testes** are the organs where **sperm** (male reproductive cells) are made. By reviewing Figure 8–4, you can identify the prostate gland.

**MIDSAGITTAL SECTION THROUGH MALE PELVIS**

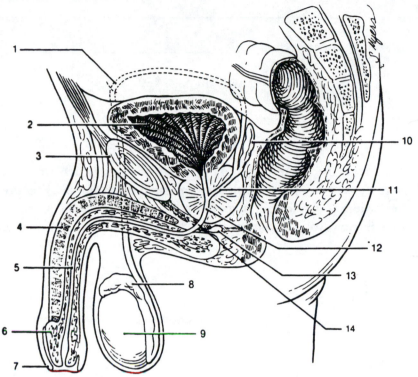

1. **Ductus vas deferens** emerging from the deep inguinal ring.

2. **Urinary bladder**

3. **Symphysis pubis**

4. **Corpus cavernosum penis**

5. **Penile urethra** seen within corpus spongiosum penis.

6. **Glans penis,** expanded end of corpus spongiosum.

7. **Prepuce,** skin which covers glans; removed in circumcision.

8. **Epididymis**

9. **Testis**

10. **Seminal vesicle**

11. **Ejaculatory duct**

12. **Prostatic urethra**

13. **Bulbourethral gland**

14. **Membranous urethra**

**Figure 8–4.** The male reproductive system. (Used with permission from Guy, J.F., *Learning Human Anatomy*, Norwalk, Conn.: Appleton & Lange, 1992.)

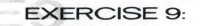

# EXERCISE 9:

What would a **prostatectomy** be? _____

(Answer on page 159)

You can also find the **ureter, urethra,** and the **rectum,** which we previously discussed. Note the **vas deferens,** which are important ducts for carrying the sperm to the urethra, where it is released. A common method of male birth control is called a **vasectomy.** By now, your medical terminology skills should allow you to define:

# EXERCISE 10:

**vasectomy** _____

_____

(Answer on page 159)

Continue with Chapter 9, The Muscular and Skeletal Systems.

# CHAPTER 8 ANSWERS

**YOUR ANSWER:   1a.**   surgical removal of the adenoids

You are incorrect. Surgical removal of the adenoids is called **adenoidectomy** (ad"e-noid-ek'to-me). Please return to page 149 and select the correct answer from the alternatives provided.

**YOUR ANSWER:   1b.**   surgical removal of a gland

You are correct. Adenectomy does refer to the surgical removal of a gland:

> **ADEN-  +  -ECTOMY  =   ADENECTOMY**
> (gland)     (to take out)      (excision of a gland)

Return to page 149.

**YOUR ANSWER:   1c.**   surgical removal of an adhesion

It was a good try, but a wrong one. An adhesion is an abnormal joining of parts to each other and is NOT managed by an adenectomy. Remember that the suffix **-lysis** refers to loosening from adhesions? Please return to page 149 and select the correct answer from the alternatives provided.

**YOUR ANSWER:   2a.**   in front of the kidneys

You are incorrect. Remember that the prefix **ad-** means to or toward or near. Return to page 149 and select another answer.

**YOUR ANSWER:   2b.**   near, on top of the kidneys

Correct. The prefix **ad-** means near, to, or toward. Therefore:

> **AD-**  =  **-REN(AL)**  =         **ADRENAL**
> (near)       (kidney)      (gland on top of the kidney)

**EXERCISE 3 ANSWERS:**

1. nephritis    *inflammation of the kidneys*
2. nephropexy    *surgical replacement of the kidney*
3. nephroma    *tumor of a kidney*
4. renointestinal    *pertaining to the kidneys and intestines*
5. nephrolithiasis    *condition of kidney stones*

**YOUR ANSWER:    4a.**    surgical incision for the removal of a stone from the renal pelvis

This is correct. The term can be broken down as follows:

**NEPHRO-** + **PYELO-** + **LITH-** + **-OTOMY** = **NEPHROPYELOLITHOTOMY**
(kidney)    (pelvis)    (stone)    (incision)    (incision to remove a stone
from the pelvis of the kidney)

See how easy it's getting to break down long terms to discern their meaning? Return to page 151.

**YOUR ANSWER:    4b.**    surgical incision into the renal pelvis

This is incorrect. There is a part of the term you have overlooked. Study the term again and continue with answer 4a. on page 151.

**EXERCISE 5 ANSWERS:**

1. cystoscope    *an instrument used to look into the urinary bladder*
2. nephrocystitis    *an inflammation of the kidneys and bladder*
3. cholecystitis    *an inflammation of the gallbladder*

**EXERCISE 6 ANSWERS:**

A **salpingo-oophorectomy** would be *a removal of the uterine tube and ovary (one or both ovaries).*

**YOUR ANSWER:    7a.**    (1) uterus pain and (2) surgical replacement of the uterus

You are incorrect. The suffix **-rrhagia** does not refer to pain. The suffix for pain is **-algia.** You are correct in defining the term **hysteropexy.** Return to page 154 and select another answer.

**YOUR ANSWER: 7b.** (1) bleeding or excessive flow from the uterus and (2) surgical puncture of the uterus

You are incorrect. You have the term **metrorrhagia** correct, but you have incorrectly defined the suffix **-pexy.** Return to page 154 and select another answer.

**YOUR ANSWER: 7c.** (1) bleeding or excessive flow from the uterus and (2) surgical replacement of the uterus

You are correct. The terms can be broken down as:

| | | | |
|---|---|---|---|
| **METRO-** + | **-RRHAGIA** | = | **METRORRHAGIA** |
| (uterus) | (excessive flow) | | (excessive flow or bleeding from the uterus) |
| **HYSTER(O)-** + | **-PEXY** | = | **HYSTEROPEXY** |
| (uterus) | (surgical fixation) | | (surgical fixation or replacement of the uterus) |

Return to page 154.

## EXERCISE 8 ANSWERS:

perinatal   *the period around the time a woman gives birth, immediately before and after*
postnatal   *after birth (refers to the newborn); postpartum is the term for the mother for the period after birth*
neonatal   *newborn (the first four weeks after birth)*

## EXERCISE 9 ANSWER:

prostatectomy   *the removal of the prostate gland (or a portion of it)*

## EXERCISE 10 ANSWER:

vasectomy   *the removal of a section of the vas deferens duct to interrupt the flow of sperm*

Continue with Chapter 9, The Muscular and Skeletal System.

# CHAPTER 8 INTERNAL SYSTEMS WORD STUDY LIST

adenectomy (ad″ĕ-nek′to-me)

adenic (ah-de′nik)

adenitis (ad″ĕ-ni′tis)

adrenal (ə-dre′nəl) gland

cholecystitis (ko″le-sis-ti′tis)

endocrine (en′do-krīn)

endometrium (en-do-me′tre-um)

excretion (eks-kre′shən)

exocrine (ek′so-krin)

genitourinary (jen″i-to-u′ri′nar-e)

hysterectomy (his″te-rek′to-me)

hysteropexy (his′ter-o-pek-se)

lymphadenitis (lim-fad″ĕ-ni′tis)

metrorrhagia (me″tro-ra′je-ah)

natal (na′təl)

neonatal (ne″o-na′təl)

nephralgia (ne-fral′je-ah)

nephritis (ne-fri′tis)

nephrocystitis (nef″ro-sis-ti′tis)

nephrolithiasis (nef″ro-li-thi′ah-sis)

nephroma (ne-fro′ma)

nephropexy (nef′ro-pek″se)

nephropyelolithotomy (nef″ro-pi″ĕ-lo-li′thot′o-me)

oophorectomy (o″of-ə-rek′tə-me)

ovaries (o′və-rez)

ovum (o′vəm)

pancreas (pan′kre-əs)

parathyroid (par″ə-thi′roid)

perinatal (per″ĭ-na′təl)

perineum (per″i-ne′um)

pituitary gland (pĭ-too′ĭtar″e)

proctoscope (prok′to-skōp)

proctoscopy (prok-tos′ko-pe)

prostatectomy (pros″tə-tek′tə-me)

pyelitis (pi″ĕ-li′tis)

rectum (rek′təm)

renal (re′nəl)

renointestinal (re″no-in-tes′ti-nal)

salpingitis (sal″pin-ji′tis)

salpingo-oophorectomy (sal-ping″-go-o″-of-o-rek′to-me)

testes (tes′tez)

thyroid (thi′roid)

ureter (u-re′ter)

urethra (u-re′thrah)

urinary (u′rĭ-nar″e)

uterus (u′tər-əs)

vagina (və-ji′nə)

vas deferens (vas de′ferens)

vasectomy (və-sek′tə-me)

vulva (vəl′və)

# chapter nine

# The Muscular and Skeletal Systems

*The body is held together and provided movement by the muscular system and the body's skeletal system. The terms associated with muscles and bones are addressed in this chapter.*

## STEM/TERM STUDY LIST

| | | |
|---|---|---|
| arthr(o)- | dactyl- | osteo- |
| cerv- | ili- | periosteum |
| chir- | ligament | spondyl(o)- |
| chondr- | my- | sterno- |
| cost- | myel- | tendon |
| crani- | | |

The muscles of the body help us move, provide support for the body, and protect nerves, blood vessels, and vital organs. Muscles can be an important part of the vital organs—such as the heart muscle and the intestinal muscles.

There are three basic types of muscles:

1. **STRIPED** (also called skeletal) **MUSCLES**—considered voluntary because we have some control over them
2. **SMOOTH MUSCLES**—involuntary muscles, such as the stomach or the pupil of the eye, since we have no direct control over their movement
3. **CARDIAC MUSCLES**—found only in the _____.

Right! Heart. The cardiac muscle is also involuntary because we cannot directly control our heartbeat.

The medical root word for muscle is **my(o)-**. The **myocardium** (mi″o-kar′-de-um) is the medical term for the heart muscle.

# EXERCISE 1:

What does **myocarditis** (mi″o-kar-di′tis) indicate?

a. an incision made into the heart muscle (page 170)
b. an inflammation of the heart muscle (page 170)

Other terms using the **my-** stem include:

**MY/OMA** (mi-o′mah)—a tumor composed of muscle tissue

**MY/ECTOMY** (mi-ek′to-me)—excision of a part of a muscle

**MY/OTOMY** (mi-ot′o-me)—dissection or incision into a muscle

## EXERCISE 2:

Define the condition **myalgia.** _____

(Answer on page 170)

Previously you learned the term **synergy** which means to work together. Muscles that work together to make a movement are called **synergists.** If these muscles fail to work together, a condition called **asynergy** occurs (notice that the prefix **a-** means "not" here.) More commonly, however, the term **ataxia** is used to describe the loss of muscle coordination. Another condition involving muscles is called **contracture** in which a muscle provides resistance to normal stretching and shortens.

Muscles are joined to bones by tough fibrous tissues called **tendons.** Tendons are so strong that they will not stretch. Between some tendons and bones are fluid-filled sacs called **bursae. Ligaments,** however, will stretch. They are the tissues that connect bone to bone.

## EXERCISE 3:

Define the following conditions:

1. tendonitis _____
2. bursitis _____

(Answer on page 170)

## EXERCISE 4:

Certain muscles have heads or points. See if you can identify how many heads the following muscles have:

1. quadriceps  _____
2. biceps  _____
3. triceps  _____

(Answers on page 170)

Additional terms you will hear in the study of muscles are **debility, atrophy,** and **dystrophy.** Debility refers to a lack or loss of strength in muscles, while atrophy is a wasting away of tissue, cells, organs, or parts of the body.

## EXERCISE 5:

From your knowledge of **dys-,** how would you define **dystrophy,** if you know that **-trophy** comes from the Greek "to nourish"?  _____

(Answer on page 170)

There are many names of muscles to be learned when studying **myology** (mi-ol'-o-je)—the science of muscles. Since this is a basic text, we won't be learning all the various names. Refer to Figures 9–1 and 9–2 for the identification of some of the most commonly used muscle names.

Our skeletal system primarily provides us with support for our body. Its rib cage and spine also help protect vital organs of the body. There are 206 bones in the adult human body. The medical root word for bone is **oste(o)-,** as used in **osteoma** (a tumor of bone tissue) and **osteomyelitis** (an inflammation of a bone, sometimes spreading and affecting the marrow [**myel-**]). You will also see the term **os** attached to the name of a bone as a descriptive term. The stem os, as in the stem osteo, means bone.

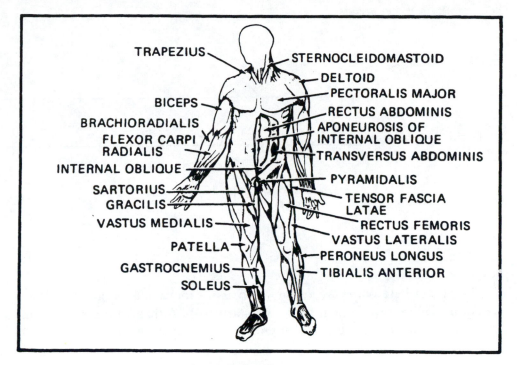

**Figure 9–1.** The muscles (anterior view)

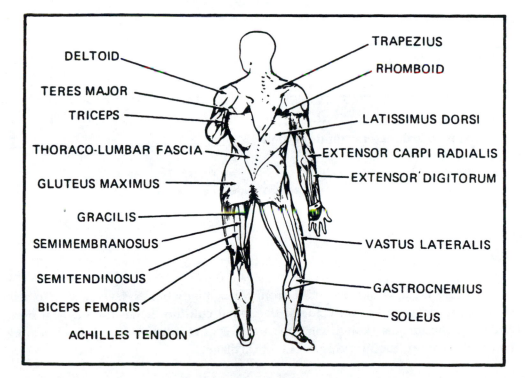

**Figure 9–2.** The muscles (posterior view)

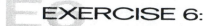EXERCISE 6:

Define **interosseous** _____

(Answer on page 171)

The place where bones are joined which allows movement is called a joint, designated in medical terminology by the stem **arthr(o)-**. **Arthritis** (ar-thri'tis) is an inflammation of the joints; **arthralgia** (ar-thral'je-ah) is a painful joint.

EXERCISE 7:

What is an **arthrectomy** (ar-threk'to-me)? _____

(Answer on page 171)

**Cartilage** is the connective tissue from which many bones develop. It also acts as a cushion between the vertebrae of the spinal column. It has the medical stem **chondr-**. A **chondroma** (kon-dro'mah) is a tumor of cartilage cells; a **chondrectomy** (kon-drek'to-me) is the surgical removal of cartilage.

# EXERCISE 8:

What is (1) **osteochondritis** (os″te-o-kon-dri′tis) and (2) **osteoarthritis** (os″te-o-ar-thri′tis)?

    a. an inflammation of bone and (1) joint and (2) cartilage (page 171)
    b. an inflammation of bone and (1) cartilage and (2) joint (page 171)

A bone has several parts to it, two of which include the marrow and the periosteum. **Marrow,** as you will learn in the discussion of the nervous system, is represented by the stem **myel(o)-.** The **periosteum** is the covering *around* the outside of the bone and is a good example of how medical terminology works:

> **PERI-** + **-OSTE(UM)** =    **PERIOSTEUM**
> (around)      (bone)      (the tough membrane
>                            that covers bone)

When a medical professional uses the term **digit** in relation to the skeletal system, it means finger or toe. **Digital** refers only to a function performed with a finger. Should a patient need a **prosthesis,** he would be fitted with an artificial part to replace a hand, arm, leg, or even a tooth.

Note in Figure 9–3 the wrist area. The term **carpal** at this point refers to the bones in this area. You may have heard of someone suffering from **carpal tunnel syndrome.** This is a set of symptoms which are concentrated in the carpal (or wrist) region.

# EXERCISE 9:

Define intercarpal _____

(Answer on page 171)

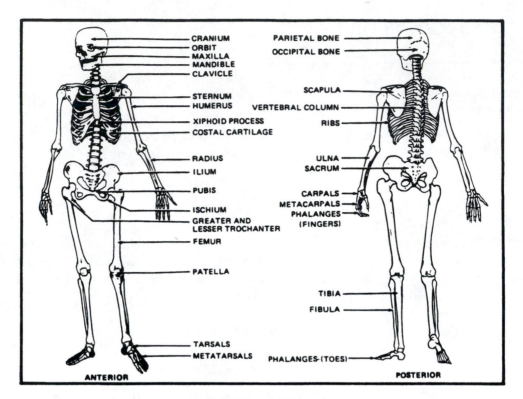

**Figure 9–3.** The skeletal system

Various areas of the body have special stems for their part of the skeleton, although not all are directly bone-related. Some of these are listed below along with examples of each.

| STEM | MEANING | EXAMPLE |
|---|---|---|
| cerv- | neck | **CERVICAL**—neck |
| | | **CERVIX**—neck of the uterus |
| chir-, cheir(o)- | hand | **CHEIROPLASTY** (ki′ro-plas′te)—plastic surgery on the hand |
| cost- | rib | **EPICOSTAL**—upon a rib |
| crani- | skull | **CRANIOTOMY**—surgery on the head |
| dactyl- | finger or toe | **DACTYLOMEGALY** (dak″ti-lo-meg′ah-le)—abnormal enlargement of fingers and toes |
| ili- | ilium (hipbone) | **ILIOSACRAL** (il″e-o-sa′kral)—pertaining to the ilium and the sacrum |

| STEM | MEANING | EXAMPLE |
|------|---------|---------|
| **spondyl(o)-** | spinal column | **SPONDYLOSYNDESIS** (spon″di-lo-sin′-de-sis)—spinal fusion |
| **stern(o)-** | sternum | **STERNAL**—relating to the sternum (breastbone) |

Continue with Chapter 10, The Nervous System.

# CHAPTER 9 ANSWERS

**YOUR ANSWER:** **1a.**  an incision made into the heart muscle

Incorrect. **-Itis** is not the suffix we learned to mean surgical incision. Return to page 162 and continue.

**YOUR ANSWER:** **1b.**  an inflammation of the heart muscle

You are correct. Myocarditis, when broken down, looks like this:

| **MYO-** | + | **CARD-** | + | **-ITIS** | = | **MYOCARDITIS** |
|----------|---|-----------|---|-----------|---|-----------------|
| (muscle) | | (heart) | | (inflammation) | | (inflammation of the heart muscle) |

Return to page 162.

## EXERCISE 2 ANSWER:

myalgia    *muscle pain*

## EXERCISE 3 ANSWER:

1. tendonitis   *inflammation of a tendon*
2. bursitis   *inflammation of a bursa*

## EXERCISE 4 ANSWERS:

1. quadriceps   *4*
2. biceps   *2*
3. triceps   *3*

## EXERCISE 5 ANSWER:

Dystrophy means *a disorder resulting from malnourishment or defective nourishment.*

## EXERCISE 6 ANSWER:

interosseus    *between bones*

## EXERCISE 7 ANSWER:

An arthrectomy is *a removal of a joint.*

**YOUR ANSWER:    8a.**   an inflammation of bone and (1) joint and (2) cartilage

You are incorrect. You have the stems for joint and cartilage reversed. Continue by studying the terms on page 166 again before selecting another answer.

**YOUR ANSWER:    8b.**   an inflammation of bone and (1) cartilage and (2) joint

You are correct. The terms mean:

| **OSTEO-** + | **CHRONDR-** + | **-ITIS** | = **OSTEOCHONDRITIS** |
|---|---|---|---|
| (bone) | (cartilage) | (inflammation of) | (inflammation of bone and cartilage) |

| **OSTEO-** + | **ARTHR-** + | **-ITIS** | = **OSTEOARTHRITIS** |
|---|---|---|---|
| (bone) | (joint) | (inflammation of) | (a degenerative joint disease that involves an inflammation of bones and joints) |

Return to page 167.

## EXERCISE 9 ANSWER:

intercarpal    *between the carpal (wrist) bones*

# CHAPTER 9 MUSCULAR AND SKELETAL SYSTEMS WORD STUDY LIST

arthralgia (ar-thral'je-ah)
arthrectomy (ar-threk'to-me)
arthritis (ar-thri'tis)
asynergy (a-sin'ər-je)
ataxia (ə-tak'se-ə)
atrophy (at'rə-fe)
biceps (bi'seps)
bursa (bər'sə)
bursitis (bər-si'tis)
cardiac (kahr'de-ak) muscles
carpal (kahr'pəl)
carpal tunnel syndrome
cartilage (kahr'tĭ-lej)
cervical (sər'vĭ-kəl)
cervix (sər'viks)
cheiroplasty (ki'ro-plas'te)
chondrectomy (kon-drek'to-me)
chondroma (kon-dro'mah)
contracture (kən-trak'chər)
craniotomy (kra"ne-ot'ə-me)
dactylomegaly (dak"ti-lo-meg'ah-le)
debility (də-bil'ĭ-te)
digit (dij'it), digital (dij'ĭtəl)
dystrophy (dis'trə-fe)
epicostal (ep"ĭ-kos'təl)
iliosacral (il"e-o-sa'kral)
intercarpal (in"tər-kahr'pəl)

interosseus (in"tər-os'e-əs)
involuntary
ligaments (lig'ə-məntz)
marrow (mar'o)
myalgia (mi-al'jə)
myectomy (mi-ek'tə-me)
myocarditis (mi"o-kar-di'tis)
myocardium (mi"o-kar'de-um)
myology (mi-ol'o-je)
myoma (mi-o'mə)
myotomy (mi-ot'ə-me)
osteoarthritis (os"te-o-ar-thri'tis)
osteochondritis (os"te-o-kon-dri'tis)
osteoma (os"te-o'mə)
osteomyelitis (os"te-o-mi"ə-li'tis)
periosteum (per"e-os'te-əm)
prosthesis (pros-the'sis)
quadriceps (kwod'rĭ-seps)
smooth muscles
spondylosyndesis (spon"di-lo-sin'de-sis)
sternal (ster'nəl)
striped muscles
synergist (sin'ər-jist)
tendonitis (ten"də-ni'tis)
tendons (ten'dən)
triceps (tri'seps)
voluntary

**10**

# The Nervous System

*Our nervous system includes the brain and spinal cord, as well as all the nerves of the body. Many of the terms you will learn in this chapter are related to the conditions and disorders that can occur within the nervous system.*

## STEM/TERM STUDY LIST

| | | |
|---|---|---|
| cephal- | encephal- | neuro- |
| cerebro- | mening- | psycho- |
| cran- | myelo- | |

The nervous system has two main divisions—**the central nervous system (CNS)** and the **peripheral nervous system (PNS)**. The central nervous system consists of the brain and spinal cord. The term **peripheral,** as you learned in earlier chapters, means around, towards the body surfaces. Therefore, the PNS runs "out" or away from the central nervous system. This is the network of nerves that go to all the outer reaches of the body from the brain and spinal cord. A part of the PNS is the **autonomic nervous system,** which controls all involuntary functions of the body such as heartbeat, intestinal contractions, and sweating.

Back to the brain—the central control center for the CNS. The brain is the control center for the nervous system. The brain is divided into four parts, commonly known as the **cerebrum** (ser′ĕ-brum), **cerebellum** (ser″ĕ-bel′um), **medulla** (mĕ-dul′ah), and **pons** (ponz). The main portion of the brain is the cerebrum, from which the stem **cerebr(o)-** comes. **Cerebro-** means the brain or relating to the brain, as in the term **cerebrovascular** (ser″ĕ-bro-vas′ku-lar)—the blood vessels of the brain. A patient who has had a **cerebrovascular accident (CVA)** has had a stroke.

## EXERCISE 1:

What is **cerebrology** (ser″ĕ-brol′o-je)?

a.  the study of strokes (page 179)
b.  the study of the brain (page 179)

Another stem for the brain is **encephal(o).** **Encephalitis** (en″sef-ah-li′tis) is an inflammation of the brain.

## EXERCISE 2:

What would an **encephaloma** (en″sef-ah-lo′mah) be?

(Answer on page 179)

Other **encephalo-** terms you may see are:

**ELECTRO/ENCEPHALO/GRAM** (elek"tro-en-sef'ah-lo-gram") **(EEG)**—a
written record of the electrical activity of the brain

**ENCEPHALO/MYEL/ITIS** (en-sef"ah-lo-mi"e-li'tis)—an inflammation of
the brain and spinal cord (myelo-)

**ENCEPHAL/ALGIA** (en-sef"ah-lal'je-ah)—pain within the head

As seen before, the stem **myel(o)-** means spinal cord. It has the more general
meaning of "pertaining to the marrow," so you sometimes will see the stem when
bones are being discussed, as marrow is the material that fills bones. **Poliomyelitis**
(po"le-o-mi"ĕ-li'tis) is an inflammation of the gray matter of the nervous system and
the spinal cord. A **myelogram** (mi'ĕ-lo-gram) is an x-ray of the spinal cord.

# EXERCISE 3:

You previously learned that the suffix **-cele** meant protrusion or swelling. What
is a **myelocele** (mi'ĕ-lo-sēl)?

a. a protrusion of the spinal cord (page 179)
b. a swelling of the brain (page 179)

The brain, of course, is found in the head. Two medical stems refer to the
head—**cephal(o)-** and **cran-**. Hydrocephalus (hi-dro-sef'ah-lus) is a condition commonly known as water on the brain. You can see that **cephal-** may sometimes also
mean brain. The **cranial** area refers to the skull.

# EXERCISE 4:

What is (1) **intracephalic** (in"trah-sĕ-fal'ik) and (2) a **craniotomy** (kra"ne-ot'-
o-me)?

a. (1) outside the head and (2) an operation on the head (page 179)
b. (1) within the head and (2) inflammation of the cranium (page 179)
c. (1) within the head and (2) an operation on the head (page 180)

The stem **neuro-** refers to nerves or the nervous system. **Neurology** (nu-rol′o-je) is the medical specialty that deals with the nervous system.

## EXERCISE 5:

From what you already know about suffixes, define the following terms that have **neur-** as the stem:

1. neurectomy (nu-rek′to-me) _____
2. neuralgia (nu-ral′je-ah) _____
3. neuroma (nu-ro′mah) _____
4. neuritis (nu-ri′tis) _____
5. neurosclerosis (nu″ro-skle-ro′sis) _____
6. subneural (səb-noo′rəl) _____

(Answers on page 180)

Covering the brain are the **meninges** (me-nin′jez)—the three membranes that cover the brain and spinal cord. These membranes are called **dura mater** (du′rah ma′ter), **pia mater** (pi′ah ma′ter), and **arachnoid** (ah-rak′noid) (see Figure 10–1). The stem that refers to this area of the nervous system is **mening(o)-**. **Meningitis** (mĕn″in-ji′tis) is a term you have probably heard. It is an inflammation of the **meningeal** (me-nin′je-al) area (the membranes surrounding the brain and spinal cord).

Medical conditions involving the nervous system and the brain include:

**AMNESIA**—the loss of memory

**PARALYSIS**—loss of or damage to motor function because of nerve damage

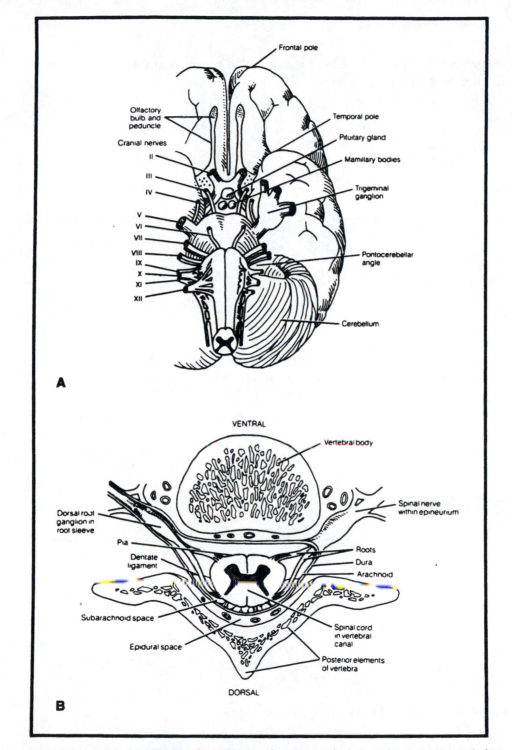

**Figure 10–1.** The brain **(A)** and spinal cord **(B).** (Reproduced with permission from DeGroot, J., Chusid, J.G. *Correlative Neuroanatomy* [20th ed.]. Norwalk, Conn.: Appleton & Lange, 1988, pp. 55, 140.)

A patient with paralysis of both legs is called a **paraplegic.** The Latin word part **-men** refers to the mind.

# EXERCISE 6:

From your previous studies, what do you think the word **dementia** (də-men′shə) means? _____

(Answer on page 180)

One last stem you should learn before leaving the nervous system refers to the mind—**psych(o). Psychology,** as you may already know, is the study of the mind and mental process. A disorder that is **psychosomatic** means it has bodily symptoms *and* emotional or mental origin. It describes anything that has to do with the mind–body relationship.

# EXERCISE 7:

From your study of suffixes, you learned **-osis.** What would **psychosis** (si-ko′sis) mean? _____

(Answer on page 180)

Continue with Chapter 11, The Respiratory System.

# CHAPTER 10 ANSWERS

**YOUR ANSWER:** **1a.** the study of strokes

You are incorrect. There is nothing in the term to indicate stroke, although strokes could be a part of the study of cerebrology, the study of the brain. Continue with the material on page 174.

**YOUR ANSWER:** **1b.** the study of the brain

Correct. **Cerebrology** is the study of the brain. Return to page 174.

**EXERCISE 2 ANSWER:**

An **encephaloma** would be a brain tumor.

**YOUR ANSWER:** **3a.** a protrusion of the spinal cord

You are correct. A **myelocele** is a protrusion of the spinal cord through the bony spinal column (see Figure 3–1, page 55). Return to page 175.

**YOUR ANSWER:** **3b.** a swelling of the brain

You are incorrect. A myelocele does not indicate a swelling of the brain. **Myel-** refers to the spinal cord. What is the stem for brain? Review the paragraph immediately before this question on page 175 and continue.

**YOUR ANSWER:** **4a.** (1) outside the head and (2) an operation on the head

You are incorrect. You need to study the prefix **intra-** again. Remember that it means within? Return to page 176 and select another answer.

**YOUR ANSWER:** **4b.** (1) within the head and (2) inflammation of the cranium

You are incorrect. Think again about the suffix **-otomy.** It does not mean an inflammation, but an incision. Return to page 176 and select another answer.

**YOUR ANSWER:   4c.**   (1) within the head and (2) an operation on the head

Correct. To verify this answer, examine the words:

| **INTRA-** | + | **-CEPHAL(IC)** | = | **INTRACEPHALIC** |
|:---:|:---:|:---:|:---:|:---:|
| (within, inside) | | (head) | | (within the head) |

| **CRANI-** | + | **-OTOMY** | = | **CRANIOTOMY** |
|:---:|:---:|:---:|:---:|:---:|
| (head) | | (surgical incision) | | (any operation on the head) |

Return to page 176.

## EXERCISE 5 ANSWERS:

1. neurectomy   *removal of a nerve*
2. neuralgia   *nerve pain*
3. neuroma   *tumor of a nerve*
4. neuritis   *inflammation of a nerve*
5. neurosclerosis   *hardening of a nerve*
6. subneural   *beneath a nerve*

## EXERCISE 6 ANSWER:

dementia   *loss of thinking abilities (involves memory, judgment, and abstract reasoning)*

## EXERCISE 7 ANSWER:

Psychosis means *a mental condition (characterized by delusions, incoherent speech, among other symptoms)*

# CHAPTER 10 NERVOUS SYSTEM WORD STUDY LIST

amnesia (am-ne′zhə)

arachnoid (ah-rak′noid)

autonomic (aw′to-nom′ik) nervous system

central nervous system (CNS)

cerebellum (ser″ĕ-bel′um)

cerebrology (ser″ĕ-brol′o-je)

cerebrovascular (ser″ĕ-bro-vas′ku-lar)

cerebrovascular accident (CVA)

cerebrum (ser′ĕ-brum)

cranial (kra′ne-əl)

craniotomy (kra″ne-ot′o-me)

dementia (də-men′shə)

dura mater (du′rah ma′ter)

electroencephalogram (EEG) (e-lek″tro-en-sef′ə-lo-gram″)

encephalalgia (en-sef″ə-lal′jə)

encephalitis (en″sef-ah-li′tis)

encephaloma (en″sef-ah-lo′mah)

encephalomyelitis (en-sef″ə-lo-mi″əli′tis)

hydrocephalus (hi-dro-sef′ah-lus)

intracephalic (in″trah-sĕ-fal′ik)

medulla (mĕ-dul′ah)

meningeal (me-nin′je-al)

meninges (me-nin′jez)

meningitis (mĕn″in-ji′tis)

myelocele (mi′ĕ-lo-sel)

myelogram (mi′ĕ-lo-gram)

neuralgia (nu-ral′je-ah)

neurectomy (nu-rek′to-me)

neuritis (nu-ri′tis)

neurology (nu-rol′o-je)

neuroma (nu-ro′mah)

neurosclerosis (nu″ro-skle-ro′sis)

paralysis (pə-ral″ĭ-sis)

paraplegic (par″ə-ple′jik)

peripheral (pə-rif′ər-əl) nervous system (PNS)

pia mater (pi′ah ma′ter)

poliomyelitis (po″le-o-mi″ĕ-li′tis)

pons (ponz)

psychology (si-kol′əje)

psychosis (si-ko′sis)

psychosomatic (si″ko-so-mat′ik)

subneural (səb-noo′rəl)

# chapter eleven

# The Respiratory System

*Our breathing mechanisms are not only in the lungs. Follow the respiratory process in Figure 11–1 as you read the material below.*

## STEM/TERM STUDY LIST

| | | |
|---|---|---|
| aer- | pharynx | pneum- |
| bronchi | pleura | trachea |
| larynx | pne- | |

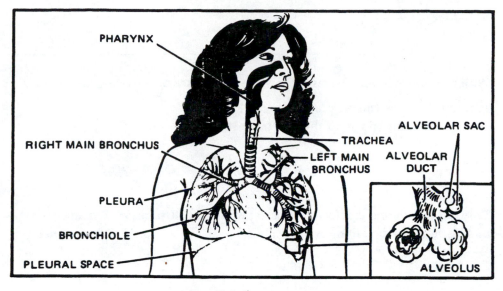

**Figure 11–1.** The respiratory system

Oxygen enters through the **nose** (nasal cavity), goes down the **pharynx** (far′inks), past the **larynx** (lar′inks) (voice box) to the **trachea** (tra′ke-ah) (also called the windpipe) to the **bronchus** (brong′kus). Oxygen enters the lung through the **bronchi,** which become smaller and smaller tubes called **bronchioles** (brong′ke-ōlz). The bronchiole then becomes an air sac called an **alveolar sac,** which contains **alveoli** (al-ve′o-li). Oxygen passes through to the bloodstream from the alveoli. This process of exchanging oxygen and carbon dioxide is called **respiration.** If the oxygen level decreases in the blood, it can cause a condition called **asphyxia.**

Each lung is protected in a sac called the **pleural sac.** The chest area of the body where the lungs are located is called the **thoracic** (tho-ras′ik) **cavity.**

The stem you will see most frequently in association with the respiratory system is **pneum(o)-,** meaning lung or air. **Pneumothorax** (nu″mo-tho′raks) is the term that means an accumulation of air in the thorax (or chest), causing the lung(s) to collapse.

Two terms can mean inflammation of the lungs—**pneumonitis** (nu″mo-ni′tis) and **pneumonia** (nu-mo′ne-ah). Pneumonia refers to the inflammation of the lungs which also are filled with a fluid or waste debris from cells. Other terms using this stem are: **pneumomycosis** (nu″mo-mi-ko′sis)—a fungus disease of the lungs, and **pneumorrhagia** (nu″mo-ra′je-ah)—hemorrhage from the lungs.

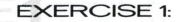

# EXERCISE 1:

Which of the following terms defines the procedure of removing lung tissue?

a. pneumectomy (nu-mek′to-me) (page 185)
b. pneumopathy (nu″mop′ah-the) (page 185)

The act of inhaling is referred to as **aspiration** or **inspiration**. Exhaling is **expiration**. The stem for breathing is **pne-**. Thus, we can have words such as **apnea** (ap-ne′ah)—not breathing.

# EXERCISE 2:

Define the following terms:

1. dyspnea (disp′ne-ah) _____
2. tachypnea (tak″ip-ne′ah) _____
3. bradypnea (brad″e-ne′ah) _____

(Answers on page 185)

One more medical stem that pertains to air is **aer(o)-**. Since only one letter changes (**e** to **i**), it should be easy to remember. **Aerobic** means filled with air; an **anaerobe** (an-a′er-ōb) is a bacteria that grows without (**an-**) free oxygen (ie, a staph infection).

Continue with Chapter 12, The Sense Organs.

# CHAPTER 11 ANSWERS

**YOUR ANSWER: 1a.** pneumectomy

Correct. **Pneumectomy** does describe the procedure of excising lung tissue.

> **PNEUM- + -ECTOMY = PNEUMECTOMY**
> (lung)  (excise)  (excision or cutting
> out of lung tissue)

Return to page 184.

**YOUR ANSWER: 1b.** pneumopathy

You are incorrect. The term you chose refers to any disease state affecting the lungs.

> **PNEUM(O)- + -PATH(Y) = PNEUMOPATHY**
> (lung)  (disease)  (lung disease)

Please return to page 184 and select the correct answer from the alternatives listed.

## EXERCISE 2 ANSWERS:

1. dyspnea  *painful, difficult breathing*
2. tachypnea  *rapid breathing*
3. bradypnea  *abnormally slow breathing*

# CHAPTER 11 WORD STUDY LIST

aerobic (ăr-o′bik)
alveolar (al-ve′ə-lər) sac
alveoli (al-ve′o-li)
anaerobe (an-a′er-ōb)
apnea (ap-ne′ah)
asphyxia (as-fik′se-ə)
aspiration (as″pĭ-ra′shən)
bradypnea (brad″e-ne′ah)
bronchi (brong′ki)
bronchioles (brong′ke-ōlz)
bronchus (brong′kus)
dyspnea (disp′ne-ah)
expiration (ek″spĭ-ra′shən)
inspiration (in″spĭ-ra-shən)

larynx (lar′inks)
nose
pharynx (far′inks)
pleural (ploor′əl) sac
pneumomycosis (nu″mo-mi-ko′sis)
pneumonia (nu-mo′ne-ah)
pneumonitis (nu″mo-ni′tis)
pneumorrhagia (nu″mo-ra′je-ah)
pneumothorax (nu″mo-tho′raks)
respiration (res″pĭ-ra′shən)
tachypnea (tak″ip-ne′ah)
thoracic (tho-ras′ik) cavity
trachea (tra′ke-ah)

# chapter twelve

# The Sense Organs

*We are all aware of the five senses: sight, sound, taste, feel, and smell. Each of these has receptors or parts of the body through which we see, hear, feel, etc. Each receptor has a medical stem that you should learn.*

## STEM/TERM STUDY LIST

aur-, aud-   lingu(o)-   ot(o)-
blephar-    olfactory   rhin-
derma-     ophthalm-

## Sight

The eye is the receptor of sight. The stem that refers to the eye is **ophthalm-.** **Ophthalmology** (of″thal-mol′o-je) is the science of the eye. The eyelid has a special stem: **blephar-. Blepharoptosis** (blef″ah-ro-to′sis) is a drooping of the upper eyelid.

## EXERCISE 1:

_____

What is (1) an **ophthalmoscope** (of-thal′mo-skōp) and (2) a **blepharoplasty** (blef′ah-ro-plas″te)?

1.  _____
2.  _____

(Answers on page 193)

## EXERCISE 2:

_____

Where is the **optic nerve?**

_____

(Answer on page 193)

Review Figure 12–1 for additional terms describing the eye itself.

## Hearing

We receive sound through our ear, also called the **auditory receptor. Aud-** and **aur-** are stems for reference to the ear. **Ot-** is also used. Your hearing is measured by an **audiometer;** an **aurist** (aw′rist) is a specialist in the diseases of the ear.

1. Pupil

2. Iris

3. Ciliary body

4. Lens

5. Choroid

6. Sclera

7. Retina

8. Optic n.

9. Cornea

10. Aqueous

11. Conjunctiva

12. Vitreous

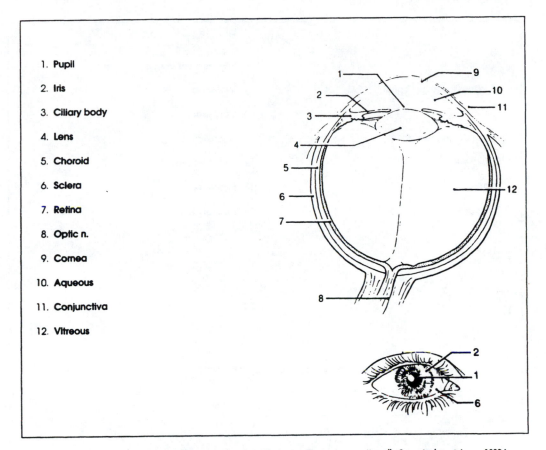

**Figure 12–1.** The right eye. (Used with permission from Guy, J.F., *Learning Human Anatomy*, Norwalk, Conn.: Appleton & Lange, 1992.)

## EXERCISE 3:

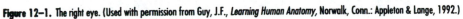

Define the following terms:

1. otoscope (o'to-skōp) _____

2. audiovisual   pertaining to the _____ and _____

1. Auricle
2. External auditory canal
3. Lobe
4. Tympanic membrane
5. Malleus
6. Incus
7. Stapes

8. Semicircular canals
9. Vestibular n.
10. Cochlear n.
11. Cochlea
12. Round window
13. Middle ear
14. Auditory tube

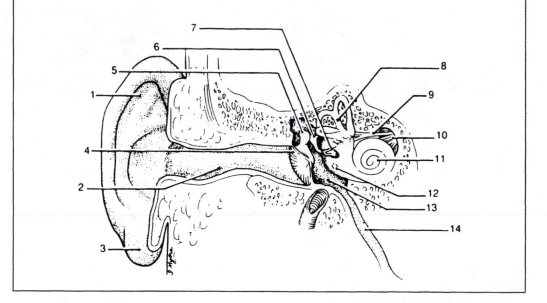

**Figure 12–2.** The right ear. (Used with permission from Guy, J.F., *Learning Human Anatomy*, Norwalk, Conn.: Appleton & Lange, 1992.)

3. otorrhagia (o"to-ra'je-ah) _____ from the _____
4. otosclerosis (o"to-skle-ro'sis) _____ of the _____

(Answers on page 193)

In Figure 12–2 you may learn more terms associated with the ear.

## Smell

We previously introduced the nasal cavity when learning the respiratory system. The medical stem used to refer to the nose is **rhin(o)-**. **Rhinoplasty** (ri'no-plas"te) is commonly called a "nose job," plastic surgery on the nose. **Olfactory** is the term which is used to refer to the sense of smell.

## EXERCISE 4:

What does **rhinopneumonitis** (ri"no-nu"mo-ni'tis) indicate?

a. inflammation of the nose and lungs (page 193)
b. inflammation of the nose and ears (page 193)
c. inflammation of the nose and throat (page 193)

You will see the term nasal pertaining to the nose, as well. A medical specialist who deals with the above senses is commonly called an **EENT** or **(ENT)**, *ey*e, *ea*r, *no*se and *th*roat specialist (or sometimes only *ea*r, *no*se and *t*hroat).

## Taste and Touch

The final two senses are taste and touch. Our tongue is the receptor for taste and is identified by the stem **lingu(o)-**. Certain medications are to be taken **sublingual**—beneath the tongue.

The touch receptor is the skin, which has the medical stem **derma-** or **dermato-**. **Dermatitis** (der"mah-ti'tis) is an inflammation of the skin. The skin is the largest organ of the body. Some medications are to be applied **topically** or on top of the skin to be absorbed by it. Other procedures are performed *percutaneously* or *through* the skin such as an injection of dye for an x-ray or a tissue biopsy.

Skin disorders may include **contusions** (bruises), **abrasions** (scratches), **cysts** (fluid-filled sacs), or **abscesses** (collections of pus).

## EXERCISE 5:

Which layer of skin is the **epidermis?**

a. the layer furthest from the top or outside (page 194)
b. the middle layer (page 194)
c. the most outside or top layer of skin (page 194)

This completes all the chapters concerned with the basics of medical terminology. From what you have learned, you should be able to break apart almost any medical term you do not know and figure out its meaning. The remaining chapters will allow you to expand on this knowledge and learn additional medical terms. GOOD LUCK!

Complete the exercise on page 196 before continuing. If you would like further practice, refer to additional exercises on pages 233–248 of the text.

# CHAPTER 12 ANSWERS

**EXERCISE 1 ANSWERS:**

1. ophthalmoscope   *an instrument used to examine the eyes*
2. blepharoplasty   *plastic surgery on the eyelid*

**EXERCISE 2 ANSWER:**

The optic nerve *goes to the eye*

**EXERCISE 3 ANSWERS:**

1. otoscope   *an instrument used to look into the ear*
2. audiovisual   *pertaining to the ears and eyes*
3. otorrhagia   *hemorrhage from the ear*
4. otosclerosis   *hardening of the (bones in the) ear*

**YOUR ANSWER:   4a.**   inflammation of the nose and lungs

You are correct. Examine the word more closely:

$$\text{RHIN(O) + PNEUM(ON) + \qquad -ITIS \qquad = RHINOPNEUMONITIS}$$

| (nose) | (lungs) | (inflammation) | (inflammation of the mucous membranes of the nose and lungs) |

Return to page 191.

**YOUR ANSWER:   4b.**   inflammation of the nose and ears

You are incorrect. Look at the stems again and return to page 191 to select another answer from the alternatives listed.

**YOUR ANSWER:   4c.**   inflammation of the nose and throat

You are incorrect. **Rhino-** does mean nose but you have incorrectly defined **pneum-**. Return to page 191 and select another answer.

**YOUR ANSWER:   5a.**   the layer furthest from the top or outside


**YOUR ANSWER:   5b.**   the middle layer

You are incorrect. Think back to our discussion of the prefix **epi-** and review it again if you need to before continuing. Then return to page 192 and select another answer from the alternatives listed.


**YOUR ANSWER:   5c.**   the most outside or top layer of skin

Correct. The prefix **epi-** means on or upon, therefore, the epidermis is the outermost layer of the skin, on top of all the rest. Return to page 192.

# CHAPTER 12 SENSE ORGANS WORD STUDY LIST

abrasions (əbra′shənz)

abscess (ab′ses)

audiometer (aw″de-om′ətər)

audiovisual

auditory (aw′dĭ-tor″e) receptor

aurist (aw′rist)

blepharoplasty (blef′ah-ro-plas″te)

blepharoptosis (blef″ah-ro-to′sis)

contusion (kən-too′zhən)

cyst (sist)

dermatitis (der″mah-ti′tis)

EENT

epidermis (ep″ĭ-dər′mis)

nasal (na′zəl)

olfactory (ol-fak′tə-re)

ophthalmology (of″thal-mol′o-je)

ophthalmoscope (of-thal′mo-skōp)

optic (op′tik)

otorrhagia (o″to-ra′je-ah)

otosclerosis (o″to-skle-ro′sis)

otoscope (o′to-skōp)

percutaneous(ly) (per″ku-ta′ne-əs)

rhinoplasty (ri′no-plas″te)

rhinopneumonitis (ri″no-nu″mo-ni′tis)

sublingual (səb-ling′gwəl)

topically

# UNIT III COMPLETION EXERCISE

Write the medical term that fits each definition below:

1. A gland that excretes into a duct _____
2. Inflammation of the gallbladder _____
3. Excessive flow from the uterus _____
4. Glands near the kidneys _____
5. The stem that refers to the lungs _____
6. Excision of a joint _____
7. Hardening of the arteries _____
8. Stem that refers to the blood vessels _____
9. Inflammation of the brain _____
10. Condition of gallstones _____

Define the following terms:

11. nephritis _____
12. cardiovascular _____
13. enterectomy _____
14. cystitis _____
15. p.c. _____
16. hepatectomy _____
17. gastroenterology _____
18. peritonitis _____
19. sublingual _____
20. bradycardia _____
21. myology _____
22. phlebitis _____
23. gastrectomy _____
24. craniotomy _____
25. hyperemesis _____

(Answers in Appendix, page 263)

# BODY SYSTEMS PUZZLE

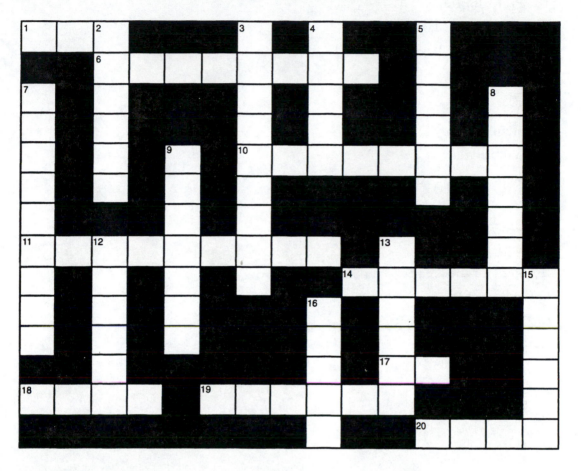

## CLUES FOR BODY SYSTEMS PUZZLE

### Across

1. Stem for ear

6. Stem for vision, eyes

10. A hormone secreted outside a gland

11. Suffix for hardening

14. Stem for the membrane surrounding the brain and spinal cord

17. Prefix for two

18. Prefix for four

19. Stem for cartilage

20. Stem for the large intestine

## Down

2. Stem for ovary

3. Gallbladder

4. Stem for sugar

5. Loss of muscle coordination

7. Upon a rib

8. Stem for lung (+-n)

9. Stem for the area between the nose and larynx

12. Tumor of fat

13. Stem for brain

15. Stem for stomach

(Answers on page 266)

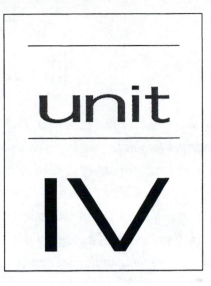

# unit
# IV

# ENLARGING YOUR MEDICAL VOCABULARY

IV

# Introduction to Unit IV

*This unit is different from the ones you have just completed. Included in this unit is more reading material and fewer exercises for you to complete. You will not find a Prefix, Suffix, or Stem/Term Study List at the beginning of any of these chapters. Instead, you should study from the Word Study List at the end of each chapter. You will be introduced to additional terms and information that will assist you in your continuing medical terminology studies. After completing this unit, you will find a group of additional exercises beginning on page 233. Take the time to complete these additional exercises before attempting the posttest.*

# chapter thirteen

# Diagnostic Terms and Tools

When a **patient (pt.)** sees a physician for the first time, the physician will want a **history and physical (H&P, Hx, or PH**—past history). During this collection of information, the health care professional will need to be informed of any medical difficulties, past surgeries, and allergic reactions to **allergens** (substances that cause reactions, such as food or pollens) or drugs.

After the history is complete, the physical examination begins with height, weight, temperature (if indicated), and blood pressure. If **febrile** pertains to fever, what would **afebrile** mean? _____ (answer on page 205.) Blood pressure is measured with a **sphygmomanometer** (also called a blood pressure cuff) and a stethoscope. The **stethoscope** will be used to listen to the blood as it returns through the arteries. It is also used to listen to sounds in the heart, lungs, intestines, fetuses, and other internal areas. A **pulse** (the expansion of an artery) is usually taken at the same time. A physician may find the patient has (1) **hypotension** or (2) **hypertension** from the sphygmomanometer results. Define those terms:

## EXERCISE 1:

(1) _____

(2) _____

(Answers on page 205)

If a patient comes to the physician with specific **symptoms (Sx),** the physician will begin listening to those in his assessment of the patient. He may need to **palpate** areas of the body to listen and feel with his hands and fingers for swelling, consistency of the area, or sounds that indicate a problem. He will ask the patient if the symptoms are **acute** (with a sudden onset) or **chronic** (continuing for a long time.) He will look for **inflammation,** changes in color, or unusual size or shape in the affected area.

The physician may decide that additional tests need to be done before a **diagnosis (Dx)** can be made. The diagnosis is the process of identifying the cause of a disease or injury. Tests are considered either **invasive** or **noninvasive.** An example of noninvasive testing is the **x-ray,** which may include a contrast agent or dye used to highlight certain areas of the body. New diagnostic tools are constantly being developed to assist the physician in an accurate diagnosis. For many years the x-ray machine has been and continues to be a valuable tool. An advanced tool to look into the body is the **computerized axial tomography (CAT or CT) scan.** It uses **radiography** (x-rays) to see and scan through the body and provide a computer view of the body in 3-D. **Magnetic resonance imaging (MRI)** is an even more advanced and safer tool to use to see what's going on within the body. In place of the harmful effects of x-rays, it uses radio waves aimed at the portion of the body to be examined. This body portion is contained in a magnetic field to absorb the radio waves. To examine and analyze the body, a computer is again used. The **ultrasound** is a test that uses sound waves to reflect back images to a monitor. It is frequently used during pregnancy to view a fetus.

Invasive tests are those which puncture the skin to get samples for further testing or insert an instrument into the body to view the affected area. Testing might involve a **biopsy (Bx),** which removes surgically a piece of tissue for further examination under a microscope. How would you classify a common blood test? Invasive _____ Noninvasive _____ (check one—answer on page 205).

Diagnostic procedures can be done either in a doctor's office, laboratory, or outpatient center of a medical center. **Ambulatory surgery** centers are being used as a way to treat a patient without a hospital stay. This can keep the costs of the treatment down in many cases. The term **ambulatory** (am"bu-lah'to"re) means to be able to walk. You will also see this term in treatments of patients as well as in diagnostic usages. Surgical patients are often urged to become ambulatory (or begin walking) as soon after surgery as possible.

There are hundreds of tests and testing devices—obviously too numerous to discuss in this text—but many involve the use of scopes **(-scopy)** and graphs **(-gram, -graphy.)** The suffix **-graphy** is often used to identify radiographic examinations (or x-rays). Try your luck at defining the following tests and tools.

# EXERCISE 2:

proctoscope _____

proctosigmoidoscope _____

cerebral arteriography _____

myelography _____

laryngoscopy _____

arthrography _____

bronchoscope _____

endoscope _____

intravenous pyelogram (IVP) _____

(Answers on page 205)

Test results may indicate the presence of a **virus** or viral infection. These are minute organisms that may cause diseases. During the diagnostic process, the **etiology** (e"te-ol'o-je) of a disease may be studied. Etiology is the study of the causes or origin of a disease. Some diseases turn out to be **idiopathic** (id"e-o-path'ik)—of unknown cause. Diseases may be **subclinical** or in their earliest stages. A **principal diagnosis** is the condition that causes a hospital admission or medical treatment. Several other diagnoses may accompany the principal diagnosis and also need to be attended to during treatment.

Immunizations are used as a **prophylactic** (protection) against diseases by injecting or inserting an **antigen** (a foreign substance) into a patient's body to produce an **antibody**—a protein substance made by the body as a response to the foreign antigen. As more and more immunizations are developed and given, more and more diseases can be eliminated or their threat greatly reduced.

Two additional terms that are not directly related to diagnostic terms but are medically important are **sterile** and **clean.** When dealing with medical patients (nonsurgical patients), the area of treatment is kept **clean,** but not necessarily sterile. The term **sterile** is used in surgical references to mean "free from living microorganisms."

If all courses of treatment fail, the patient may succumb to the symptoms and die. Additional diagnostic tests might be performed in the course of an **autopsy.** **Postmortem** (_____ death) examinations give clues and insights into causes of a patient's death by examining tissues, cells, blood samples, stomach contents, and skin condition just to name a few.

Diagnostic terms are abundant. From your previous studies of the body systems, you should be able to figure out the area of the body being examined along with the type of examination. At this point, study the word list at the end of the chapter before continuing to Chapter 14, Surgical Terms and Tools.

# CHAPTER 13 ANSWERS

**Page 201:**

afebrile   *not feverish, without fever*

## EXERCISE 1 ANSWERS:

hypotension   *low blood pressure*
hypertension   *above normal blood pressure*

**Page 202:**

A common blood test is *invasive*—it punctures the skin.

## EXERCISE 2 ANSWERS:

proctoscope   *an instrument used to examine the rectum*
proctosigmoidoscope   *an instrument used to examine the rectum and colon*
cerebral arteriography   *a test to see the arteries in the brain*
myelography   *an x-ray examination of the spinal cord*
laryngoscopy   *an examination into the larynx*
arthrography   *an x-ray exam of a joint*
bronchoscope   *an instrument used to look into the bronchi*
endoscope   *an instrument to look inside an internal, hollow organ*
intravenous pyelogram (IVP)   *an insertion of a dye into the renal pelvis to examine it by x-ray*

postmortem   *after death*

# CHAPTER 13 DIAGNOSTIC TERMS AND TOOLS WORD STUDY LIST

acute (ə'kut')

afebrile (a-feb'ril)

allergens (al'ər-jen)

ambulatory (am'bu-lah'to"re)

antigen (an'tĭ-jen)

arthrography (ahr-throg'rə-fe)

autopsy (aw-top'se)

biopsy (Bx) (bi'ŏp-se)

bronchoscope (brong'ko-skōp)

cerebral arteriography (sə-re'brəl ahr"tĕr-e-og'rə-fe)

chronic (kron'ik)

clean

computerized axial tomography (CAT or CT) scan

diagnosis (Dx) (di"əg-no'sis)

endoscope (en'do-skōp)

etiology (e"te-ol'o-je)

history and physical (H&P, Hx, or PH—past history)

idiopathic (id"e-o-path'ik)

immunization (im"u-nĭ-za'shən)

intravenous pyelogram (IVP) (in"trə-ve'nəs pi"ə-lo-gram)

laryngoscopy (lar"ing-gos'kə-pe)

magnetic resonance imaging (MRI)

myelography (mi"ə-log'rə-fe)

palpate (pal'pāt)

patient (pt.)

postmortem (post-mor'təm)

principal diagnosis

proctoscope (prok'to-skōp)

proctosigmoidoscope (prok"to-sig-moid'o-skōp)

prophylactic (pro"fə-lak'tik)

pulse

sphygmomanometer (sfig"mo-mə-nom'ə-tər)

sterile (ster'il)

stethoscope (steth'o-skōp)

subclinical

symptom (Sx) (simp'təm)

ultrasound (ul'trə-sound)

viral (vi'rəl)

virus (vi'rəs)

x-ray

# chapter fourteen

# Surgical Terms and Tools

In the previous chapter, you learned that one method of diagnosis, the biopsy, is usually a surgical procedure. You have also been introduced to surgical suffixes that identify the type of surgical procedure being done. Keep in mind that not all surgeries are done in a hospital requiring overnight stays.

For a period of time prior to surgery, a patient must be **NPO** (nothing by mouth) to prevent regurgitating and damaging newly placed sutures and tender tissues. Before a surgery can begin, the patient needs to be administered **anesthesia** (something to cause the loss of feeling). Anesthetics may cause various reactions, including nausea. It may be local—affecting only a small area—or general—affecting the entire body. To administer a general anesthetic, a patient will be **intubated.** In other words, an **endotracheal** tube will be inserted to keep the airway open.

## EXERCISE 1:

Where is the **endotracheal tube** placed? _____

(Answer on page 213)

I.V. lines are also started to be able to keep fluids going and provide a path for blood transfusions and insertion of medications, if needed.

The most commonly used tool in surgery is the **scalpel,** a knife used to make an **incision** (cut) (see Fig. 14–1).

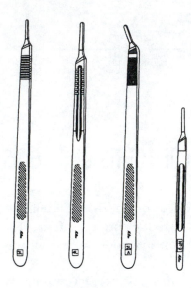

Scapel Blade Handles

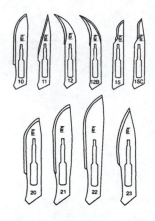

Blades

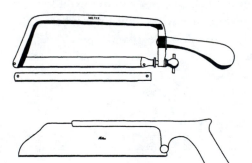

Bone Saws

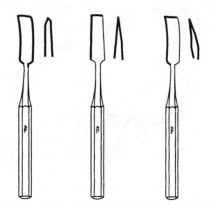

Osteotomes

**Figure 14–1.** Scalpels, bone cutter, osteotome

Surgical blades come in various sizes and degrees of thickness, depending on the size and type of incision needed. The blade handle may also vary depending on what the instrument is being used to do. A disposable blade attaches to it. Also used for cutting are various types of scissors, saws, and **osteotomes.**

# EXERCISE 2:

What does an **osteotome** cut into? _____

(Answer on page 213)

Scissors are used to cut both tissue and sutures (stitches.) These instruments are all classified as "sharps."

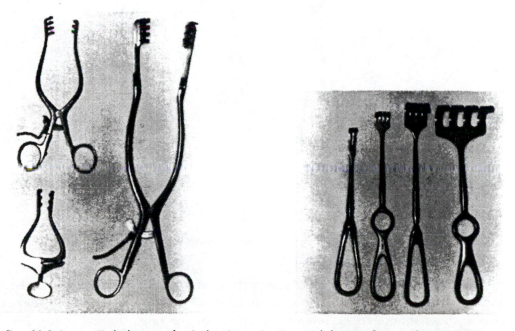

**Figure 14–2.** Retractors. (Used with permission from Groah, L., *Operating Room Nursing,* 2nd edition. Norwalk, Conn.: Appleton & Lange, 1990.)

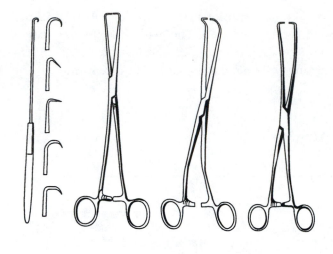

Tenaculum

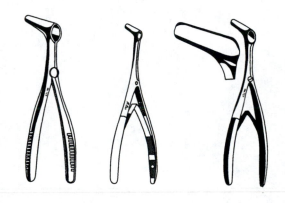

Speculum

**Figure 14–3.** Tenaculum, speculum

Several types of surgical instruments are used to hold and grasp tissue. **Retractors** hold back organs and tissue and the edges of a wound so that a surgeon can work without interference. Some retractors resemble rakes, as you see in Figure 14–2. **Tenacula** (Figure 14–3) are instruments with a hooked end used to grab and

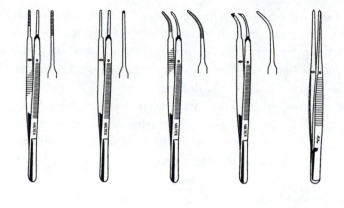

Forceps

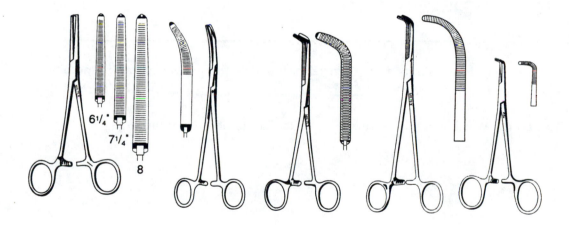

Hemostats

Figure 14–4. Forceps and hemostats

hold tissues but can also be used to pierce organs for removal or testing. **Forceps** likewise grasp and hold tissue, but they frequently have no teeth to prevent damage to the tissue or organ. **Sponge forceps** are primarily used to hold gauze pads to absorb excess fluids as needed. This group of clamping instruments also includes the **hemostat** (Figure 14–4). Can you determine what this does from your knowledge so far? If you identified it as an instrument that stops the flow of blood, you are correct. The grasping ends of clamping instruments have small ridges to prevent slipping. Surgical tools are delivered to the operating room in sterile packs that contain the instruments needed for the particular kind of surgery the patient requires.

Surgery can be small and delicate, even requiring the use of microscopes for **microsurgery.** On a different scale, highly intensified light beams called **lasers** are becoming common as surgical instruments because there is a more direct application and less bleeding occurs. Laser surgery is often used to repair eye disorders.

## EXERCISE 3:

On occasion, a surgeon or physician will decide the patient has an inoperable condition. Define inoperable. _____ (Answer on page 213)

Review the Word Study List at the end of this chapter before continuing.

# CHAPTER 14 ANSWERS

**EXERCISE 1:**

An endotracheal tube is placed *inside the trachea (windpipe)*

**EXERCISE 2:**

An osteotome *cuts into bone*

**EXERCISE 3:**

inoperable    *not able to be operated on*

# CHAPTER 14 SURGICAL TERMS AND TOOLS WORD STUDY LIST

anesthesia (an″es-the′ze-ah)

blade handle

endotracheal (en″do-tra′ke-al)

forceps (for′seps)

general

hemostat (he′mo-stat)

I.V.

incision (in-sizh′ən)

inoperable (in-op′ər-ə-bəl)

intubate (in′too-bāt)

laser (la′zər)

local

microsurgery (mi′kro-sər″jər-e)

NPO

osteotome (os″te-o-tom″)

retractor (re-trak′tor)

scalpel (skal′pəl)

sharps

sponge forceps

surgical blades

suture (soo′chər)

tenaculum (tenacula), (tə-nak′u-ləm)

# chapter fifteen

# Pharmacology Terms

**Pharmacology** is the study of drugs, their effects and reactions on the body, and their proper dosages. Along with a few terms to help in your medical studies, you will find two listings of abbreviations frequently seen in this area of study.

All legal prescription drugs in the United States are controlled by the **FDA (Food and Drug Administration).** These drugs go through extensive research and testing to be considered safe for human patients and are designated for a particular diagnosis. The study of a drug's effect on the body over a period of time is called **pharmacokinetics.** It takes into account the amount of the drug present in the blood, tissues, and body wastes and what happens because of it. The pharmacist is the health care professional licensed to sell, dispense, and prepare drugs according to the physician's prescription. **OTC (over-the-counter)** drugs are those available for public purchase without a prescription. Oftentimes, previous prescription-only drugs will become OTC after many years of usage with minimal complications and side effects.

Drugs come in a variety of categories from the "antis" such as anti-inflammatory, antibiotic, and antihistamines to the *de*congestants, muscle relaxants, and hormonal drugs. The purpose of a drug can often be seen in its categorical name. We often only know drugs by their brand name. It is the generic name given to a drug when it is developed that is often just as important to learn. For instance, we know Tylenol but we may not know acetaminophen, the generic name.

One other type of "medication" you may see charted is the **placebo.** This is a medical treatment or prescription given more for the psychological benefit of the patient than the medicinal benefit. Placebos are not harmful and are also given as part of a clinical study to patients designated as the "control" group.

It is important, as you are aware, that correct dosages and times of medications are followed. Study and learn the abbreviations below associated with times and preparations of medications. Most health care facilities also print their own "approved" list of abbreviations. The ones provided here are the most commonly used and may vary from those with which you need to become familiar.

*Abbreviations Used According to Time and Hour of Administration*

| ABBREVIATION | MEANING |
| --- | --- |
| a.c. | before food or meals |
| ad lib. | as desired |
| alt. hor. | alternate hours, every other hour |
| A.M. | before noon |
| b.i.d. | two times a day |
| h. | hour |
| h.s. | at bedtime, hour of sleep |
| n. or noc. | night |
| p.c. | after food or meals |
| P.M. | after noon |
| p.r.n. | as necessary, as required |
| q. | every |
| q.d. | every day |
| q.o.d. | every other day |
| q.h. | every hour |
| q.i.d. | four times a day |
| q2h | every 2 hours (use with any number) |
| stat. | immediately, at once |
| t.i.d. | three times a day |

*Abbreviations Used According to Preparation and Administration*

| ABBREVIATION | MEANING |
|---|---|
| aa | of each |
| ad | up to |
| agit. | shake, stir |
| amp. | ampule |
| aq. | water |
| bib. | drink |
| C. | centigrade |
| c̄ | with |
| cap. | capsule |
| cc | cubic centimeter |
| cm | centimeter |
| comp. | compound |
| dil. | dilute |
| dim. | one-half |
| disp. | dispense |
| div. | divide |
| dr. | dram |
| elix. | elixir |
| ext. | extract |
| F. | Fahrenheit |
| fld., fl. | fluid |
| Gm. | gram, grams |
| gr. | grain, grains |
| gtt., gtts | drop, drops |
| hypo., H. | hypodermically |
| id. | the same |
| I.M. | intramuscularly |
| I.V. | intravenously |

| ABBREVIATION | MEANING |
| --- | --- |
| **lb.** | pound |
| **lin.** | liniment |
| **liq.** | liquid |
| **lot.** | lotion |
| **m.** | minim |
| **mEq** | milliequivalent |
| **oz.** | ounce |
| **p̄** | after |
| **per** | by |
| **p.o.** | by mouth |
| **qns** | quantity not sufficient |
| **q.s.** | a sufficient quantity |
| **qt.** | quart |
| **s̄** | without |
| **s.c., subQ, S.Q.** | subcutaneously, under the skin |
| **sol.** | solution |
| **ss** | one-half |
| **syr.** | syrup |
| **tab.** | tablet |
| **tbsp.** | tablespoonful |
| **tr., tinct.** | tincture |
| **tsp.** | teaspoonful |

# CHAPTER 15 PHARMACOLOGY TERM STUDY LIST

FDA
generic (jənər′ik)
OTC
pharmacist (fahr′mə-sist)

pharmacology (fahr″mə-kol′ə-je)
pharmacokinetics (fahr″mə-ko-ki-net′iks)
placebo (plə-se′bo)

# Oncology Terms

Another medical specialty that seems to be growing in importance is the field of **oncology,** which deals with tumors. Tumors can be either **benign** (slow-growing, non-cancerous) or **malignant** (fast-growing, cancerous, life-threatening). The term **neoplasm** refers to a new abnormal growth, such as a tumor.

It is the malignant tumors that are called **cancer.** They can be caused by **carcinogens** (known cancer-causing substances such as asbestos and tobacco) or **oncogenes** (genes that cause normal cells to turn cancerous).

**Metastasis** is the term in cancer that means cancerous cells have moved and spread from one part of the body to a distant part through the bloodstream or lymph system. By now you have learned that the suffix **-oma** means tumor. Cancer has three types of categories:

**Carcinomas**—tumors of epithelial cells

**Sarcomas**—tumors of connective cells

**Mixed cancers**—combinations of both types of cells are involved in the tumor

## EXERCISE 1:

Identify these types of cancer:

osteosarcoma _____

hypernephroma _____

myeloma _____

liposarcoma _____

(Answers on page 222)

Courses of therapy to treat cancerous tumors include **chemotherapy, radiation therapy,** and surgery. Chemotherapy is the use of cancer-fighting chemicals and drugs. It is occasionally used in conjunction with radiation therapy, the use of concentrated x-rays aimed at the tumor to kill the diseased cells. These procedures are done by health care professionals trained in **nuclear medicine.** It may even be necessary to use internal radiation therapy by implanting radioactive material near the cancerous tumor.

With the best course of treatment or combination of treatments, a patient may go into **remission,** where the disease (cancer) symptoms are diminishing.

New therapies and alternative treatments are coming into focus daily, creating new terms along with them. This is not only happening in oncology, but throughout the medical field. As you continue your studies, the prefixes, suffixes, stems, and terms you have learned here should guide you to the meanings of even more complex terminology.

Continue with Chapter 17, Medical Financial Terms, to complete your introductory studies.

# CHAPTER 16 ANSWERS

## EXERCISE 1 ANSWERS:

osteosarcoma   *a malignant tumor in a bone composed of connective tissue*

hypernephroma   *a cancerous tumor in the kidney area*

myeloma   *a tumor found in bone marrow and composed of those cells*

liposarcoma   *a malignant tumor composed of fat cells*

# CHAPTER 16 ONCOLOGY TERMS STUDY LIST

benign (be-nīn')
carcinogen (kahr-sin'ə-jən)
carcinoma (kahr"si-no'mə)
chemotherapy (ke"mo-ther'ə-pe)
hypernephroma (hi"pər-nə-fro'mə)
liposarcoma (lip"o-sahr-ko'mə)
malignant (mə-lig'nənt)
metastasis (mə-tas'tə-sis)
mixed cancer
myeloma (mi"ə-lo'mə)

neoplasm (ne'o-plz-əm)
nuclear (noo'kle-ər) medicine
oncogene (ong'kō-jen)
oncology (ong-kol'ə-je)
osteosarcoma (os"te-o-sahr-ko'mə)
radiation (ra"de-a'shən) therapy
remission (re-mish'ən)
sarcoma (sahr-ko'mə)
tumor

# chapter seventeen 17

# Medical Financial Terms

The health insurance and billing field has become more and more complex over the past few years. Governmental regulations have added terms and abbreviations that did not exist in the medical field a short time ago. More new restrictions and ways of dealing with them are confronting medical office personnel. New **reimbursement** ideas are being created as well, in attempts to stem the skyrocketing costs of health care. Managed health care is commonly being used by reimbursement organizations today.

**Reimbursement organizations** are those that pay or **reimburse** the health care provider for the medical treatment of the patient. Many types of reimbursement organizations exist. Insurance companies (such as Blue Cross/Blue Shield) are the most common, but even they have various reimbursement options employers or individuals can choose. Another term for the reimbursement organization is **third-party payer.** In other words, the payment of the bill comes from someone other than the patient.

One option reimbursement organizations offer is called a **preferred provider organization (PPO).** If a patient receives treatment from a preferred provider, the reimbursement organization will pay for more of the bill. The preferred provider has an agreement with the reimbursement organization to accept the payment the organization makes. Patients who receive treatment from nonpreferred providers will probably end up paying more of the bill from their own pockets.

A **health maintenance organization (HMO)** differs from the insurance company reimbursement organization in that it collects the payment for health care (usually on a monthly basis) *and* provides the care or approval for the care that is provided. The health maintenance organization manages and/or operates doctors' clinics and labs. Specialized and hospital care is contracted out. The doctors work for the HMO, rather than operate their own offices. Some reimbursement organizations offer their own HMO but the patient has a **primary care physician** selected from an approved list provided by the HMO. The reimbursement organization does not actually operate a clinic or lab. The primary care physician directs and approves all care for the patient and refers the patient to other approved physicians for specialized care. The location where the care is given is called **point of service (P.O.S.)**

An **individual practice association (IPA)** is a type of HMO in which a patient pays a set monthly fee for health care coverage but sees his or her primary care physician in the physician's own office. The physician must be from a selected list and must approve all the care the patient receives. The physician has a contract with the IPA to provide this care but may also see patients with other health care plans. A newer type of HMO plan, called an **open HMO,** allows the patient to choose a higher **deductible** (explained below) if that patient chooses not to go to an HMO physician.

Both reimbursement organizations and HMOs may require the patient to pay a **deductible** or **co-pay** before the HMO or third-party payer begins to pay. The amount of the deductible will vary according to the health care plan the patient has chosen. A **prospective payment** is the amount the health care provider can expect to receive in payment for services provided. It is a flat rate for anyone with a particular illness, injury, or condition no matter what it may have cost the provider to give the care.

All medical illnesses, injuries, and conditions have been divided into **diagnostic-related groups (DRGs)**. DRGs have been gathered together to fit into **Major Diagnostic Categories (MDCs)**. There are over 460 DRGs and twenty-three MDC groupings. The DRGs were derived from the **International Classification of Diagnoses,** 9th edition **(ICD-9-CM)**. ICD-9 is a comprehensive list of over 8,000 possible diagnoses that have been agreed upon by the members of the World Health Organization. An updated version of diagnoses is expected out in the year 2000. Hospitals, health care agencies, and reimbursement organizations use the code number assigned to the diagnosis for their records. For a complete listing of DRGs, see the Additional Resources section at the end of this text.

The government agency that regulates health care in the United States is the **Department of Health and Human Services (DHHS).** It administers the Medicare and Medicaid programs, as well as Social Security and other social programs funded by the Federal government. Medicare and Medicaid are types of reimbursement organizations. The **Health Care Financing Administration (HCFA)** is the agency that is directly responsible for monitoring the Medicare program within the Department of Health and Human Services. Each state has set up a **peer review organization (PRO)** to monitor the physicians and the quality of care given to Medicare patients.

The complexities of the medical finance system are many and constantly changing. It is hoped that this introduction to some of the terms used will benefit you as you continue your study in the medical field.

# CHAPTER 17 MEDICAL FINANCIAL WORD STUDY LIST

co-pay
deductible
Department of Health and Human Services (DHHS)
diagnostic-related groups (DRGs)
Health Care Financing Administration (HCFA)
health maintenance organization (HMO)
individual practice association (IPA)
International Classification of Diagnoses, 9th ed. (ICD-9)

Major Diagnostic Categories (MDCs)
managed health care
open HMO
peer review organization (PRO)
point of service (POS)
preferred provider organization (PPO)
primary care physician
prospective payment
reimbursement
reimbursement organization
third-party payer

# chapter eighteen

# Additional Medical Abbreviations and Symbols

The following charts should assist you in learning even more medical abbreviations and symbols. The abbreviations introduced in the text have not all been included here. See the Index if you are looking for a specific abbreviation and cannot find it in this listing or the listings from Chapter 15. At the end of this information, you will find an exercise for Unit IV. Complete this exercise to review the information presented to you in this unit. You may also wish to work through the additional exercises presented to you before attempting the Posttest, which begins on page 249.

| ABBREVIATION | MEANING |
| --- | --- |
| abd | abdomen |
| ADL | activities of daily living |
| AIDS | acquired immune deficiency syndrome |
| A.M.A. | American Medical Association |
| AMA | against medical advice |
| ant. | anterior |
| ASAP | as soon as possible |
| ASHD | arteriosclerotic heart disease |
| BM | bowel movement |
| BMR | basal metabolic rate |
| BP | blood pressure |
| Bx | biopsy |
| CA | cancer |
| CAD | coronary artery disease |
| CBC | complete blood count |

| ABBREVIATION | MEANING |
|---|---|
| CC | chief complaint |
| CCU | cardiac (or coronary) care unit |
| CHD | coronary heart disease or congenital heart disease |
| CHF | congestive heart failure |
| Chol | cholesterol |
| CNS | central nervous system |
| COPD | chronic obstructive pulmonary disease |
| CPR | cardiopulmonary resuscitation |
| C.S. | central supply |
| CV | cardiovascular |
| CVA | cerebrovascular accident (stroke) |
| CXR | chest x-ray |
| D&C | dilation and curettage |
| DC | discontinue |
| Dx | diagnosis |
| ECG, EKG | electrocardiogram |
| EEG | electroencephalogram |
| EMG | electromyogram |
| ENT | ear, nose, and throat |
| ER, ED | emergency room, emergency department |
| FBS | fasting blood sugar |
| FH | family history |
| Fx | fracture |
| GA | general anesthesia |
| GI | gastrointestinal |
| GU | genitourinary |
| GYN | gynecology |
| Hb, Hgb | hemoglobin |
| H&P | history and physical |

| ABBREVIATION | MEANING |
| --- | --- |
| **HHD** | hypertensive heart disease |
| **HOB** | head of bed |
| **Hx** | history |
| **ICU** | intensive care unit |
| **I & O** | intake and output |
| **IVP** | intravenous pyelogram |
| **IPPB** | intermittent positive pressure breathing |
| **Ⓛ** | left |
| **LMP** | last menstrual period |
| **MI** | myocardial infarction (heart attack) |
| **MS** | multiple sclerosis |
| **NG** | nasogastric |
| **NPO** | nothing by mouth |
| **NSAID** | nonsteroidal anti-inflammatory drug |
| **N & V** | nausea and vomiting |
| **OOB** | out of bed |
| **OPD** | outpatient department |
| **OR** | operating room |
| **OT** | occupational therapy |
| **OTC** | over the counter (drug) |
| **PERLA (PERRLA)** | pupils equal and reactive to light and accommodation (pupils equal, round, and reactive to light and accommodation) |
| **pt.** | patient |
| **PT** | physical therapy |
| **PTA** | prior to admission |
| **Px** | prognosis |
| **Ⓡ** | right |
| **rbc** | red blood cell |
| **RBC** | red blood cell count |

| ABBREVIATION | MEANING |
| --- | --- |
| R.N. | registered nurse |
| R/O | rule out |
| ROM | range of motion |
| R.R. | recovery room, respiratory rate |
| R.T. | respiratory therapy, radiation therapy |
| Rx | treatment |
| SICU | surgical intensive care unit |
| SOB | shortness of breath |
| STD | sexually transmitted disease |
| Sx | symptom |
| T | temperature |
| TPR | temperature, pulse, and respiration |
| Tx | traction, treatment |
| ua | urinalysis |
| WBC | white blood cell count |
| wt. | weight |
| YO | year old |
| YOB | year of birth |

## Medical Symbols

| SYMBOL | MEANING |
| --- | --- |
| – | negative |
| + | positive |
| Δ | change |
| × | times |
| ∅ | nothing |
| @ | at |
| ↑ | increasing, high |
| ↓ | decreasing, low |

| SYMBOL | MEANING |
|--------|---------|
| = | equals |
| ♀ | female |
| ♂ | male |
| > | greater than |
| < | less than |

# UNIT IV EXERCISE

Define the following terms and abbreviations:

1. etiology _____
2. benign _____
3. sterile _____
4. diagnosis _____
5. sphygmomanometer _____
6 Bx _____
7. virus _____
8. ambulatory _____
9. MRI _____
10. pt _____
11. endotracheal _____
12. intubate _____
13. IV _____
14. sharps _____
15. hemostat _____
16. sponge forceps _____
17. malignant _____
18. p.c. _____
19. t.i.d. _____
20. p.o. _____
21. carcinoma _____
22. oncology _____
23. remission _____
24. deductible _____
25. reimbursement _____
26. primary care physician _____
27. HMO _____
28. CAT scan _____
29. chronic _____
30. clean _____

(Answers on page 266)

# ADDITIONAL EXERCISES

If you feel you still need practice with the medical terms presented in the text before you attempt the Posttest, work the following exercises. Answers begin on page 267 in the Appendix.

Watch your spelling carefully!

# ABBREVIATION EXERCISE 1:

Write the definition of the abbreviation in the space provided.

1. s̄ _____
2. ENT _____
3. CVA _____
4. I.V. _____
5. TPR _____
6. R.R. _____
7. b.i.d. _____
8. NPO _____
9. pt. _____
10. Rx _____
11. C.V. _____
12. I.M. _____
13. c̄ _____
14. I & O _____
15. EKG _____
16. t.i.d. _____
17. CA _____
18. O.R. _____
19. B.P. _____
20. ua _____
21. p.r.n. _____

22. h.s. _____
23. H & P _____
24. CBC _____
25. stat _____

(Answers on page 267)

# ABBREVIATION EXERCISE 2:

Define the following abbreviations:

1. I & O _____
2. spec. _____
3. c̄ _____
4. PERLA _____
5. p.c. _____
6. ENT _____
7. D & C _____
8. IPPB _____
9. H & P _____
10. CVA _____
11. gtts _____
12. pt. _____
13. Fx _____
14. q4h _____
15. ℞ _____
16. a.c. _____
17. I.V. _____
18. h.s. _____
19. CNS _____
20. cc _____
21. Tx _____
22. C.V. _____
23. ml _____
24. Bx _____
25. noc. _____

(Answers on page 268)

# ADDITIONAL EXERCISE 1:

Write the medical term that fits each definition:

1. Excessive sensitivity to pain _____
2. Against or counter to bacteria _____
3. Blood poisoning _____
4. The outer layer of skin _____
5. Painful urination _____
6. Too much blood sugar _____
7. Removal of a part of the intestines _____
8. Hardening of the arteries _____
9. What you place at the beginning of a word to further its meaning _____
10. The system of vessels that do not carry blood _____
11. Abnormally slow heartbeat _____
12. External secretion _____
13. Inflammation of the gallbladder _____
14. Abnormal stoppage of menstruation _____
15. A condition involving the white blood cells _____
16. Science of the stomach and intestines _____
17. Inflammation of a nerve _____
18. Glands on top of the kidneys _____
19. Inflamed condition of the brain _____
20. A minute arterial branch _____
21. Situated upon a rib _____
22. The terminal portion of the small intestine _____
23. Stem that refers to the blood vessels _____
24. Excision of a joint _____
25. Without pain _____

Define the following terms and word elements:

26. electrocardiogram _____
27. epinephrine _____
28. suffix _____
29. albuminuria _____
30. endoparasite _____
31. cystitis _____
32. ab- _____

33. a.c. _____
34. arthrocele _____
35. epi- _____
36. dermatitis _____
37. ilium _____
38. cholelithiasis _____
39. asepsis _____
40. ana- _____
41. -oma _____
42. anaerobe _____
43. enterocentesis _____
44. cardiovascular _____
45. aden- _____
46. abortion _____
47. -em(ia) _____
48. enteradenitis _____
49. alb- _____
50. arthritis _____

(Answers on page 269)

# ADDITIONAL EXERCISE 2:

_____

Fill in the definition of each word:

1. peripheral _____
2. supine _____
3. hyperglycemia _____
4. enterocentesis _____
5. septicemia _____
6. ventral _____
7. prone _____
8. cholecystitis _____
9. arteriole _____
10. amenorrhea _____
11. adduction _____
12. inferior _____
13. exocrine _____
14. ostectomy _____

15. epidermis _____

16. hyperalgesia _____

17. leukemia _____

18. lateral _____

19. adrenal _____

20. pyemia _____

21. epicostal _____

22. ileum _____

23. dorsal _____

24. encephalitis _____

25. sagittal _____

_____

(Answers on page 270)

# ADDITIONAL EXERCISE 3:

_____

Mark the prefix (P), root word (R), suffix (S) and define the following words.

(*Example:* phleb/itis    *inflammation of a vein*)

(R)    (S)

1. colostomy _____

2. hyperadiposis _____

3. myoma _____

4. ostemia _____

5. endocarditis _____

6. arthrectomy _____

7. arteritis _____

8. dermatitis _____

9. hypotension _____

10. intrahepatic _____

11. retrosternal _____

12. preoperative _____

13. neuroplasty _____

14. quadriplegia _____

15. dyspnea _____

(Answers on page 271)

# ADDITIONAL EXERCISE 4:

Define the following terms:

1. lateral _____
2. enteritis _____
3. hypoglycemia _____
4. intravenous _____
5. nephrocystitis _____
6. craniotomy _____
7. supine _____
8. bradycardia _____
9. post mortem _____
10. colostomy _____
11. encephalitis _____
12. endocarditis _____
13. ventral _____
14. arthritis _____
15. hyperthermia _____
16. hepatopexy _____
17. gastroscope _____
18. hemiplegia _____
19. dyspnea _____
20. appendectomy _____
21. phlebitis _____
22. retropleural _____

23. hemostat _____
24. neurology _____
25. arteriosclerosis _____

Define the following prefixes:

26. a-, an- _____
27. exo- _____
28. epi- _____
29. retro- _____
30. hyper- _____
31. intra- _____
32. peri- _____
33. anti- _____
34. dys- _____
35. hypo- _____

Define the following suffixes:

36. -itis _____
37. -ectomy _____
38. -otomy _____
39. -emia _____
40. -plasty _____

Define the following stems:

41. chole- _____
42. cardi- _____
43. aden- _____
44. hepat- _____
45. arthr- _____

Define the following abbreviations:

46. b.i.d. _____
47. q4h _____
48. h.s. _____
49. I & O _____
50. ua _____

(Answers on page 272)

## Crossword Puzzle 5

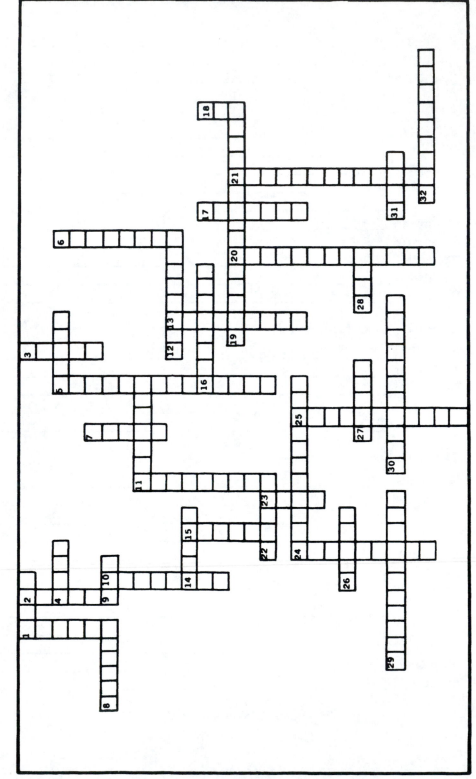

# Clues for Crossword Puzzle 5

## ACROSS

1. The basic body or component of a word
4. Within, inside
5. Word element meaning bile
8. Placed at the beginning of a word
9. Stem meaning kidneys
11. Prefix for arteries
12. Word meaning before birth
14. Stem denoting blood
16. Inflammation of the urinary bladder
19. Medical term for kidney stones
22. Suffix for condition of
24. The membranous sac that surrounds the heart
26. The prefix meaning lung
27. The prefix meaning rapid
28. The prefix meaning under or below
29. Cutting out or removal of the whole or part of the stomach
30. Before the onset of fever
31. Prefix meaning many or much
32. Abnormal slowness of breathing

## DOWN

1. Placed at the end of a word
2. Word element for electrical or electricity
3. Suffix for cut or incision
5. Word that means the body's system of heart, arteries, veins, and capillaries
6. Pertaining to the neck
7. The prefix meaning above, beyond, or extreme
10. Stem denoting the head and brain
11. Inflammation of the joints
13. The outer layer of the skin
15. Reduced number of red blood cells
17. A tumor or mass of bony tissue
18. The prefix for bad, improper, painful
20. The study of the eye and its diseases

21. Situated between two muscles
23. The suffix denoting inflammation
24. Inflammation of vein
25. Situated within the vein or veins

(Answers on page 274)

# CASE HISTORY #1

Below you will find a case study. Obviously, this is a fictitious patient with several complications. This study will give you an opportunity to review a patient's records as you might see it written in the health care setting. Additional information is usually added to a patient's chart—this is only the highlights with the medical terms for you. See if you can define the underlined terms on the answer sheet provided at the end of the case history. The answers may be found on page 275.

# BEST CARE HOSPITAL

Anytown, USA

Patient: Baga, Ruta          Room No.                    Type:

Hospital No. 00-00-00        Dictating: Wilma Flintstone, M.D.

Admit Date 00/00/95          Attending:

                             Referring:

# REASON FOR ADMISSION:

This is one of multiple admissions for this 60-year-old woman admitted with a problem of increasing **(1) abdominal** pain for the past seven days.

# HISTORY OF PRESENT ILLNESS:

For the past seven days, the patient has had increasing mid to lower abdominal pain. This is fairly steady, severe, worse with walking, twisting, turning. It was very severe when her dog jumped on her abdomen several times. She has had a low-grade fever to 100°F, no chills or sweats. She has had slightly loose stools, no blood, no **(2) anorectal** discomfort. A urinalysis yesterday showed *Klebsiella* urine with bacteria and culture pending. She was seen this morning as an outpatient and admitted because of persistent pain, tenderness, and guarding in the lower abdomen.

## PREVIOUS HOSPITALIZATIONS:

The patient was admitted to BCH from the **(3) ED.** She entered with acute nausea and vomiting at the time, and she was drinking heavily—a bottle of wine or more daily. She also was smoking several packs of cigarettes daily. **(4) Endoscopy** by Dr. Blue showed severe **(5) esophagitis** and **(6) gastritis,** believed related to alcohol, but with no definite ulcers and no **(7) gastrointestinal** bleeding. At that time she had a white count of 3.3, hemoglobin 11.7, hematocrit 34.2, with an MCV of 104. Liver chemistries included an albumin of 3.2, ALT 62, AST 77, bilirubin 0.6, alkaline phosphatase 108, GTP 663. Ultrasound showed a fatty liver. The patient recovered uneventfully. In the last year or so, the patient reports that she has decreased her use of alcohol significantly.

## MEDICAL HISTORY:

History otherwise shows no indication of large bowel disease, diverticulitis, or IBD. Significant illnesses include frequent urinary tract infections without evidence of obstructive **(8) uropathy.** She is subject to migraine headaches recurrent since age 18 and occurring two or three per month and then skipping for some months. Her major problem has been a mood disorder for many years, probably bipolar, dominantly depressed. She has been seeing Dr. Green, a psychologist, twice a week, and she sees a psychiatrist periodically for medications. Medications listed below.

## SURGICAL HISTORY:

1. Ruptured ectopic pregnancy age 40, explored, and the tube was removed.
2. Repair of posttraumatic left ulnar nerve with scar tissue removal and a Z-plasty at age 27 with good functional result.

## ALLERGIES:

None defined.

## FAMILY HISTORY:

Nothing known about her father who left when she was age 15. The mother, living at age 85, has had bladder cancer with multiple recurrences since age 60. She has three siblings and two sisters, three of whom are half-siblings.

## CURRENT MEDICATIONS:

1. Anafranil 50 **(9) mg** 5 x **(10) q.d.** for depression prescribed by Dr. Green
2. Lithium 450 mg twice daily, recently started
3. Klonopin 0.5 mg 1 **(11) t.i.d.** with meals and 2 to 4 at bedtime for sleep
4. Xanax 0.25 **(12) p.r.n.**
5. Codeine for migraine headaches p.r.n.

## PHYSICAL EXAMINATION:

Vital signs: Pulse 86; blood pressure 120/80; temperature 98°F

## GENERAL APPEARANCE:

Uncomfortable-appearing woman complaining of abdominal pain

## ASSESSMENT:

1. Probable acute diverticulitis
2. Irritated bladder with possible urinary tract infection, probably secondary to acute diverticulitis
3. Depression, bipolar, on lithium
4. Heavy consumption of alcohol, long-standing, with previous fatty liver demonstrated and macrocytic **(13) anemia**
5. Previous alcohol-related gastritis and esophagitis, June 1993
6. Left ulnar nerve with Z-plasty removal of scar tissue
7. History of post-motor vehicle accident, left ulnar nerve injury, age 27, repaired at the Mayo Clinic
8. Recurrent migraine headaches since age 18

9. Ruptured tubal pregnancy, explored at age 40
10. **(14) Chronic** abuse of cigarettes since age 18

## COMMENT AND PLAN:

The patient has been experiencing acute lower abdominal pain and now has guarding and rebound probably secondary to acute diverticulitis. She has numerous associated medical conditions as noted above including severe bipolar depression disease, currently on lithium. Management will be as follows:

1. Clear fluids
2. **(15) IV rehydration**
3. Metronidazole 750 mg **(16) q6h** loading dose and 500 q8h
4. Rocephin 2 gm I.V. **(17) q24h**
5. Demerol 75 mg for pain along with Vistaril 25 mg **(18) I.M.**
6. Continue her usual psychiatric medications as listed above
7. Consider flexible **(19) sigmoidoscopy** and Gastrografin enema in the morning
8. Antacids to be given **(20) p.c.**

## WRITE YOUR ANSWERS HERE:

1. abdominal _____
2. anorectal _____
3. ED _____
4. endoscopy _____
5. esophagitis _____
6. gastritis _____
7. gastrointestinal _____
8. uropathy _____
9. mg _____
10. q.d. _____
11. t.i.d. _____
12. p.r.n. _____
13. anemia _____
14. chronic _____
15. IV rehydration _____

16. q6h _____

17. q24h _____

18. I.M. _____

19. sigmoidoscopy _____

20. p.c. _____

## DISCHARGE SUMMARY:

Now, try your luck at the underlined words in this medical record. Once again, you will find an answer sheet at the end and the answers are on page 275.

## BIGG MEDICAL CENTER

Small Town, USA

| | | |
|---|---|---|
| Patient: | Cane, Candy | |
| Hospital No.: | 99-99-99 | |
| Admit Date: | 00/00/95 | Dictating: I. M. Good, M.D. |
| Discharge Date: | 00/03/95 | Attending: |
| | | Referring: |

## HISTORY OF PRESENT ILLNESS:

This was the second Bigg Medical Center admission for this 73-year-old diabetic woman with **(1) malignant (2) hypertension** and severe azotemia, who had failed to appear for follow-up after discharge from the hospital about a year ago. For further details, one is referred to the admission history and physical examination.

## LABORATORY RESULTS:

Hematocrit 30.9, **(3) WBC** 9200 with a normal differential. Chemistry panel showed a low $CO_2$ of 18, sugar of 146, BUN of 51, creatinine 4.6, albumin 3.0, iron 32, cholesterol 261. Creatinine clearance with a creatinine of 5.8, calculated to only 8 ml. Urinalysis positive for occult blood, 100 mg percent of protein and 2 to 5 white blood cells. The protein quantization amounted to 2772 mg.

Chest x-ray showed **(4) cardiomegaly** with congestive heart failure, **(5) pleural** effusion and interstitial edema. **(6) Renal** ultrasound showed small kidneys with moderate cortical thinning but no **(7) hydronephrosis.** **(8) Electrocardiogram** was abnormal with sinus rhythm, ST-T wave abnormalities and prolonged Q-T interval.

## HOSPITAL COURSE:

The patient was essentially admitted with malignant hypertension with her initial blood pressure in the emergency room having been 260/160. The patient was placed in **(9) ICU** and started on diuretics and Nipride, and had improvement of her blood pressure followed by a progressive rise in her creatinine. Within 48 hours her blood pressure had improved to 155/70. Funduscopic examination showed **(10) bilateral** flame-shaped **(11) hemorrhages,** as well as status post-bilateral laser treatment. The patient was felt to be in a malignant, accelerated phase of her diabetic **(12) nephropathy** and close to a dialysis level. The patient had very little insight into her illness and was difficult to communicate with at times, being quite reluctant to have studies carried out. Her blood pressure was purposely kept in a range above 140 to avoid further decline of her renal function. The patient was started on Epogen because of hematocrit falling below 30 by 2/23/95.

On 2/24/95, because of the significant edema and azotemia, she was started on hemodialysis after a Vas-catheter was inserted. The patient tolerated dialysis very well. Her blood pressure became easier to control, utilizing Procardia-XL predominantly.

The patient also received iron. Minoxidil for better blood pressure control was added on 2/26/95 but subsequently was discontinued.

The patient underwent insertion of a left forearm Gore-tex shunt. The patient was in stable and satisfactory condition on 3/3/95 and was discharged.

## WRITE YOUR ANSWERS HERE:

1. malignant _____
2. hypertension _____
3. WBC _____
4. cardiomegaly _____
5. pleural _____
6. renal _____
7. hydronephrosis _____
8. electrocardiogram _____

9. ICU _____

10. bilateral _____

11. hemorrhage _____

12. nephropathy _____

# POSTTEST

1. In a medical term, the **prefix** comes _____before_____
   A. before the stem
   B. after the stem
   C. either of the above
2. The three parts of a medical term are the **prefix, stem, and** _____suffix_____
   A. compound
   B. combining form
   C. suffix
3. The term **retrosternal** means _____behind to    breastbone_____
   A. behind the breastbone
   B. to the left of the breastbone
   C. to the right of the breastbone
4. **Subcutaneous means** _____beneath the skin_____
   A. adjacent to the skin
   B. beneath the skin
   C. within the skin
5. **Preoperative** refers to which part of a surgical procedure _____
   _____
   A. the time period before the operation
   B. the recovery period after the operation
   C. the period during the operation
6. A medication given **p.c.** is given _____
   A. before a meal
   B. at noon
   C. after a meal
7. **Postmortem** means _____
   A. before death
   B. after death
   C. causing death

# MATCHING

Choose the word or words in Column B that describe the prefix, stem, or suffix listed in Column A. Some of the definitions in Column B may be used more than once.

|  | **A** |  | **B** |
|---|---|---|---|
| 8. | Epi- *n* | a. | eye |
| 9. | Endo- *G* | b. | liver |
| 10. | Osteo- *J* | c. | intestine |
| 11. | Myo- | d. | wall of a structure |
| 12. | Arthro- *l* | e. | blood |
| 13. | Phlebo- *P* | f. | ear |
| 14. | Stoma- | g. | within, inside |
| 15. | Encephalo- | h. | kidney |
| 16. | Entero- | i. | muscle |
| 17. | Hyper- | j. | bone |
| 18. | Hypo- | k. | vein |
| 19. | Oto- *A* | l. | joint |
| 20. | -emia *E* | m. | spinal cord |
| 21. | Mono- *X* | n. | on, upon |
| 22. | Myelo- | o. | below or low |
| 23. | Nephro- | p. | artery |
| 24. | Reni- | q. | mouth |
| 25. | Arterio- | r. | skin |
| 26. | Hepato- | s. | midline |
| 27. | Hemo- | t. | around |
|  |  | u. | brain |
|  |  | v. | posterior |
|  |  | w. | above or |
|  |  | x. | one |

28. The term **anesthesia** means _____.
    A. without sensation
    B. heightened sensitivity
    C. excruciating pain
29. A preparation used to counteract a poison is called an _____.
    A. antipyretic
    B. antialexic
    C. antidote
30. The term **intravenous** means _____.
    A. within a cell
    B. beneath a cell
    C. outside a cell
31. **Extracellular** means _____.
    A. within a cell
    B. beneath a cell
    C. outside a cell
32. **Leukocyte** refers to a _____ blood cell.
33. **Erythrocyte** refers to a _____ blood cell.
34. An **abductor** muscle is one which moves a body part _____ the midline.
35. The word **anteroposterior** would be translated as from _____ to back.
36. **Latero-** refers to the _____ of an object or body.
37. **Hydrocephalus** means water in the _____.
38. **Dysuria** describes _____.
39. **Nocturia** refers to a condition characterized by excessive urination during the _____.
40. One or more letters or syllables at the beginning of a word, which explains or adds to the meaning of the rest of the term, is called a _____.
41. **Polyuria** is a condition characterized by _____ urination.
42. **Leukopenia** is a blood disorder characterized by too _____ leukocytes.
43. **Dermatosclerosis** describes a condition that involves the _____ of the skin.
44. **Aphagia** is a condition which is characterized by the inability to _____.
45. The term **appendectomy** describes the surgical _____ of the appendix.
46. The main body or basic component of a word is called the _____.
47. **Lymphadenopathy** refers to a disease of the lymph _____.
48. **Dermatomyositis** describes an infection of the _____ and the muscles.
49. **Arthritis** refers to an inflammation of a _____.

50. **Myocarditis** describes a condition characterized by inflammation of the _____ muscle.

51. **Pneumonitis** refers to inflammation of the _____.

52. A **sphygmomanometer** measures _____.

53. The term **gastroscope** describes an instrument used to look into the _____.

54. A person suffering from a disease characterized by **polyuria** would void _____.

55. **Monomorphic** means having which form or shape? _____
    A. a single form or shape
    B. many forms or shapes
    C. an unsual form or shape

56. The term **bicuspid** refers to a structure which has _____.
    A. a single point or cusp
    B. two points or cusps
    C. three or more points or cusps

57. In the term **triangle,** the prefix **tri-** indicates _____.
    A. one
    B. two
    C. three

58. How many letters are found in a word described as a **tetragram?** _____
    A. two
    B. three
    C. four

59. **Multicellular** means composed of _____.
    A. one cell
    B. few cells
    C. many cells

60. **Hemiplegia** describes a condition in which there is _____.
    A. paralysis of one lateral half of the body
    B. paralysis of both sides of the body
    C. paralysis of the upper half of the body

61. The medical term **pericardium** means _____.
    A. around the heart
    B. within the heart
    C. adjacent to the heart

62. Which of the following terms means between the ribs? _____
    A. intracostal
    B. infracostal
    C. intercostal

63. Which two of the following prefixes may be used to mean white in medical terms? _____
    **A.** alb-
    **B.** alge-
    **C.** leuk-

64. In the term **bradycardia,** the prefix **brady-** means _____.
    **A.** sporadic
    **B.** slow
    **C.** rapid

65. The condition characterized by a fast heartbeat is called _____.
    **A.** bradycardia
    **B.** arrhythmia
    **C.** tachycardia

66. **Hypotension** refers to _____.
    **A.** elevated blood pressure
    **B.** low blood pressure
    **C.** absence of blood pressure

67. **Hypertension** refers to _____.
    **A.** elevated blood pressure
    **B.** low blood pressure
    **C.** absence of blood pressure

68. **Hyperglycemia** refers to _____ sugar in the blood.

69. _____ is the science and study of the brain.

70. A patient who is lying face down and flat is in a _____ position.

71. A muscle tumor is called a _____.

72. **Nephritis** means inflammation of the _____.

73. The abbreviation for the word that means a needle shot into a muscle is _____.

74. In surgery, the suffix _____ means to form, build up, or repair.

75. A swelling in the tissue that contains fluid is indicated by the suffix _____ .

76. The position in which the body and its parts are lying on their dorsal or back surfaces is called _____.

77. The term used to refer to the tail end of the body is _____.

78. The excision of a portion of the colon (or the whole colon) is called a _____.

79. Formation of an artificial opening into the colon is called a _____.

80. **Cystocele** describes a hernial _____ of the urinary bladder.

81. **Cystotomy** describes a surgical _____ into the bladder.

82. The excision of part of the intestine is known as an _____.

83. Inflammation of the stomach is known as _____.

84. **Hepatitis** refers to an infection which is centered in the _____.
85. **Nephrolithiasis** indicates a condition commonly known as _____ stone or stones.
86. In a medical term, the stem **chole-** refers to _____.
87. The term **hematuria** refers to _____ in the urine.
88. **Lipoma** refers to a tumor which is composed of _____ tissue.
89. **Cholelithiasis** describes a disease state characterized by the presence of gall _____.
90. Used in a medical term, the stem **reni-** refers to the _____.
91. **Neuritis** describes inflammation of a _____.
92. **Osteoarthritis** refers to inflammation of _____ and _____.
93. **Phlebitis** means inflammation of a _____.
94. A letter or syllable placed at the end of a word to add to its meaning is called a _____.
95. The term **hepatoma** describes a _____ of the liver.
96. **Lymphadenitis** refers to a condition characterized by inflammation or _____ of the lymph glands.
97. **Hydrarthrosis** describes a disease characterized by the presence of water in a _____.
98. **Hematemesis** describes a condition characterized by the _____ of blood.
99. Instruments used to cut, saw, or make an incision are classified as _____.
100. The science and study of tumors is called _____.

(Answers begin on page 276)

# APPENDIX

**ANSWERS TO:**

## Pretest Solutions

(Answers to pages ix–xv)

1. c. suffix
2. a. before the stem
3. b. within a vein
4. c. outside a cell
5. a. behind the breastbone
6. b. beneath the skin
7. a. around the heart
8. c. intercostal
9. c. ante mortem
10. a. the time period before the operation
11. b. after death
12. a. without sensation
13. c. antidote
14. a. a single form or shape
15. b. two points or cusps
16. c. three
17. c. four
18. c. many cells
19. c. a large quantity of urine
20. a. paralysis of one lateral half of the body
21. a. elevated blood pressure
22. b. low blood pressure
23. c. tachycardia

24. b. slow
25. a. alb-
26. white
27. red
28. toward
29. front
30. side
31. water
32. painful
33. loss
34. prefix
35. stem or root
36. glands
37. skin
38. joint
39. heart
40. lungs
41. heart
42. stomach
43. liver
44. kidney
45. bile, gallbladder
46. blood
47. fat or fatty
48. stones
49. kidneys
50. nerve
51. bone
52. vein
53. suffix
54. tumor
55. infection
56. science, study
57. vomiting
58. myocarditis
59. pneumonitis
60. much or frequent
61. few
62. skin

63. eat, swallow
64. removal
65. colectomy
66. colostomy
67. protrusion
68. incision
69. enterectomy
70. gastritis
71. an excess of
72. before
73. deficiency
74. myoma
75. kidney
76. removal
77. -plasty
78. -cele
79. supine
80. caudal
81. n
82. g
83. j
84. i
85. l
86. k
87. f
88. e
89. x
90. t
91. h
92. e
93. b
94. p
95. h
96. o
97. w
98. c
99. u
100. q

# Unit I

## Prefix Exercise

(Answers to page 47)

The following prefixes from Column A are matched with the definition in Column B. Some definitions have been used more than once.

| | **A** | | **B** |
|---|---|---|---|
| 1. a- | D | | A. slow |
| 2. endo- | F | | B. between |
| 3. anti- | N | | C. above, excessive |
| 4. hypo- | K | | D. without, not |
| 5. tachy- | L | | E. bad |
| 6. mal- | E | | F. within, inside |
| 7. intra- | F | | G. backwards |
| 8. ante- | I | | H. on, upon |
| 9. hyper- | C | | I. before |
| 10. exo- | O | | J. together |
| 11. epi- | H | | K. below, beneath |
| 12. retro- | G | | L. fast |
| 13. dys- | E | | M. near |
| 14. inter- | B | | N. against |
| 15. an- | D | | O. out, away from |

(Answers to puzzle on page 48)

# PREFIX PUZZLE

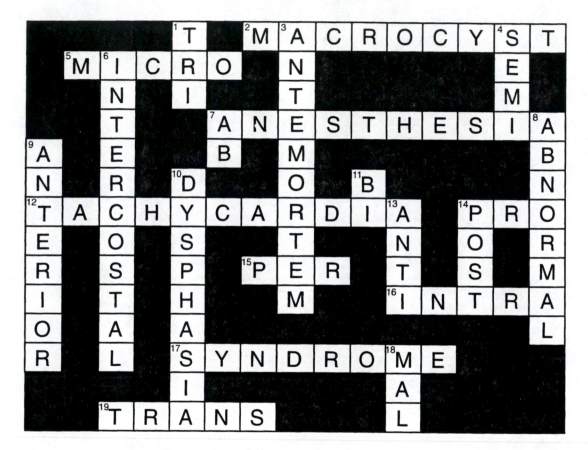

## Unit II Suffix Exercise

(Answers to page 79)

Definitions of the following terms are:

1. gastralgia    *pain in the stomach*
2. arthralgia    *pain in a joint*

3. anemia    *low level of red blood cells in the blood (without blood)*
4. dermatitis    *inflammation of the skin*
5. gastrectomy    *removal of all or part of the stomach*
6. pneumectomy    *removal of all or part of a lung*
7. neurology    *the science and study of the nerves, nervous system*
8. tracheotomy    *surgical incision in the trachea (windpipe)*
9. leukemia    *a condition involving the white blood cells*
10. esophagoscopy    *an examination of the esophagus*
11. nephropexy    *surgical repair (fixation) of a kidney*
12. splenopexy    *surgical replacement of a displaced spleen*
13. neuroplasty    *surgical repair of a nerve*
14. blepharoplasty    *surgical repair of the eyelid*
15. cardiology    *the science and study of the heart and its diseases*
16. dermatology    *the study of the skin and its diseases*
17. arthritis    *inflammation of a joint*
18. suffix    *element placed at the end of a word to further its meaning*
19. cholelithiasis    *condition of gallstones*
20. colostomy    *creation of an artificial opening into the colon*

The medical term that the definition describes is:

1. Inflammation of the heart    *carditis*
2. Excision or removal of a joint    *arthrectomy*
3. Inflammation of the brain    *encephalitis*
4. Science of the stomach and intestines    *gastroenterology*
5. Blood poisoning    *septicemia (pyemia)*
6. A surgical puncture of the intestines    *enterocentesis*
7. Removal of stones from the kidney    *nephrolithotomy*
8. A tumor of a muscle    *myoma*
9. The suffix that means to create an artificial opening or mouth    *-ostomy*
10. Procedure used to look into the bladder    *cystoscopy*

(Answers to puzzle on page 81)

# SUFFIX PUZZLE

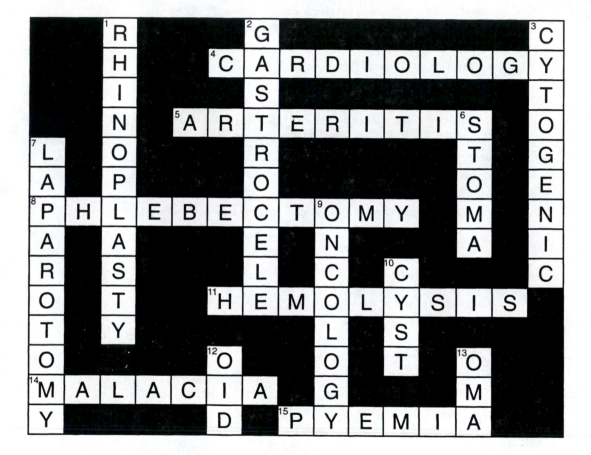

## Unit III

## Completion Exercise

(Answers to page 196)

The medical term that fits each definition is:

1. A gland that excretes into a duct   *exocrine*
2. Inflammation of the gallbladder   *cholecystitis*
3. Excessive flow from the uterus   *metorrhagia*
4. Gland near the kidneys   *adrenal*
5. The stem that refers to the lungs   *pneum(o)-*
6. Excision of a joint   *arthrectomy*
7. Hardening of the arteries   *arteriosclerosis*
8. Stem that refers to the blood vessels   *vascular*
9. Inflammation of the brain   *encephalitis*
10. Condition of gallstones   *cholelithiasis*

The definitions of the following terms are:

11. nephritis   *inflammation of the kidneys*
12. cardiovascular   *system of heart, arteries, veins, and capillaries*
13. enterectomy   *surgical removal of part of the intestines*
14. cystitis   *inflammation of urinary bladder*
15. p.c.   *after meals*
16. hepatectomy   *surgical removal of part of the liver*
17. gastroenterology   *science and study of stomach and intestines*
18. peritonitis   *inflammation of peritoneum (lining of the abdomen)*
19. sublingual   *beneath the tongue*
20. bradycardia   *abnormally slow heart beat*
21. myology   *science and study of the muscles*
22. phlebitis   *inflammation of a vein*
23. gastrectomy   *surgical removal of all or part of the stomach*
24. craniotomy   *an operation on the head*
25. hyperemesis   *excessive vomiting*

## Anatomical Postures

(Answers to page 121)

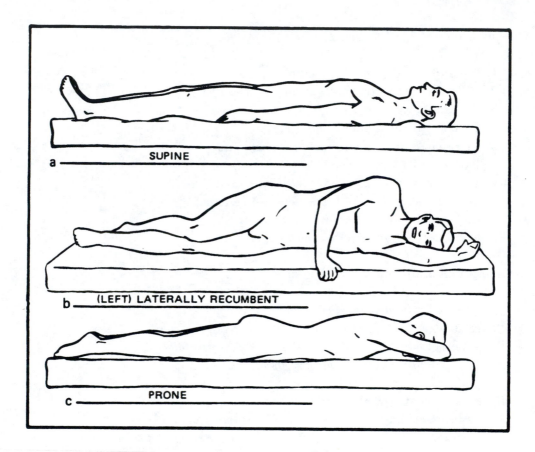

a _____ SUPINE _____

b _____ (LEFT) LATERALLY RECUMBENT _____

c _____ PRONE _____

# Body Locations and Positions

(Answers to puzzle on page 122)

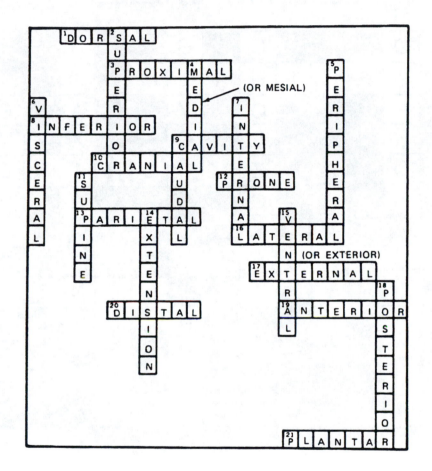

(Answers to puzzle on page 197)

# BODY SYSTEMS PUZZLE

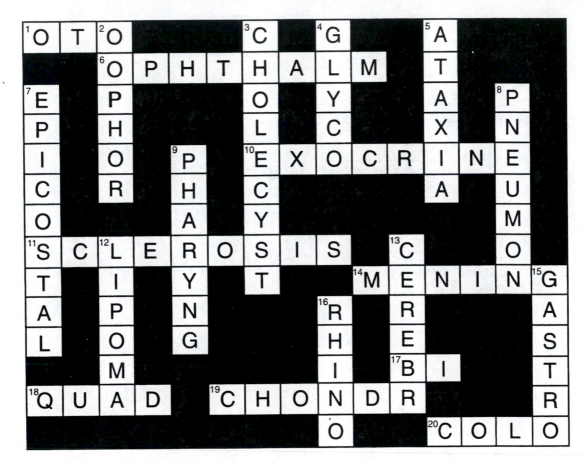

## Unit IV Exercise Answers

(Answers to page 232)

1. etiology    *the study of causes or origin of a disease*
2. benign    *not harmful; chances for recovery are good*
3. sterile    *free from living microorganisms*
4. diagnosis    *identification of the cause of a disease or injury*
5. sphygmomanometer    *instrument used to measure blood pressure*

6. Bx   *biopsy*
7. virus   *minute organisms which may cause a disease*
8. ambulatory   *able to walk*
9. MRI   *magnetic resonance imaging*
10. pt   *patient*
11. endotracheal   *within the trachea (windpipe)*
12. intubate   *insertion of a tube to keep the airway open*
13. IV   *intravenous*
14. sharps   *surgical instruments used to cut bone, tissue, or sutures*
15. hemostat   *instrument used to stop the flow of blood*
16. sponge forceps   *instrument used to hold gauze pads during surgery to absorb fluids*
17. malignant   *harmful, lethal, life-threatening*
18. p.c.   *after meals*
19. t.i.d.   *three times a day*
20. p.o.   *by mouth*
21. carcinoma   *a tumor made up of epithelial cells*
22. oncology   *study of tumors*
23. remission   *period when disease symptoms diminish*
24. deductible   *amount paid before the health insurance begins payment*
25. reimbursement   *the payment back to someone for services*
26. primary care physician   *physician through which all of a patient's care is channeled*
27. HMO   *health maintenance organization*
28. CAT scan   *computerized axial tomography; instrument used to provide a 3-D view of the body*
29. chronic   *continuing for a long time*
30. clean   *reference to medical (nonsurgical) patient's area of treatment; not necessarily completely free of living microorganisms*

# ADDITIONAL EXERCISE ANSWERS
## Abbreviation Exercise 1 Answers

(Answers to page 233)

The definitions of the abbreviations are:

1. s̄   *without*
2. ENT   *ear, nose, and throat*
3. CVA   *cerebrovascular accident (stroke)*

4. I.V.   *intravenous*

5. TPR   *temperature, pulse, and respiration*

6. R.R.   *recovery room*

7. b.i.d.   *twice a day*

8. NPO   *nothing by mouth*

9. pt.   *patient*

10. Rx   *therapy, treatment, prescription*

11. C.V.   *cardiovascular*

12. I.M.   *intramuscular*

13. c̄   *with*

14. I&O   *intake and output*

15. EKG   *electrocardiograph (or gram)*

16. t.i.d.   *three times a day*

17. CA   *cancer*

18. O.R.   *operating room*

19. B.P.   *blood pressure*

20. ua   *urinalysis*

21. p.r.n.   *as needed*

22. h.s.   *at bedtime, hour of sleep*

23. H&P   *history and physical*

24. CBC   *complete blood count*

25. stat   *immediately*

# Abbreviation Exercise 2 Answers

(Answers to page 234)

Definitions of the abbreviations are:

1. I&O   *intake and output*

2. spec.   *specimen*

3. c̄   *with*

4. PERLA   *pupils equal and reactive to light and accommodation*

5. p.c.   *after meals*

6. ENT   *ear, nose, throat*

7. D & C   *dilation and curettage*

8. IPPB   *intermittent positive pressure breathing*

9. H&P   *history and physical*

10. CVA   *cerebrovascular accident (stroke)*

11. gtts   *drops*

12. pt.   *patient*

13. Fx    *fracture*
14. q4h    *every four hours*
15. Ⓡ    *right*
16. a.c.    *before meals*
17. I.V.    *intravenous*
18. h.s.    *hour of sleep, bedtime*
19. CNS    *central nervous system*
20. cc    *cubic centimeter*
21. Tx    *traction*
22. C.V.    *cardiovascular*
23. ml    *milliliter*
24. Bx    *biopsy*
25. noc.    *night*

# Additional Exercise 1

(Answers to page 235)

The medical term that fits each definition is:

1. Excessive sensitivity to pain    *hyperalgesia*
2. Against or counter to bacteria    *antibacterial*
3. Blood poisoning    *septicemia (or pyemia)*
4. The outer layer of skin    *epidermis*
5. Painful urination    *dysuria*
6. Too much blood sugar    *hyperglycemia*
7. Removal of a part of the intestines    *enterectomy*
8. Hardening of the arteries    *arteriosclerosis*
9. What you place at the beginning of a word to further its meaning    *prefix*
10. The system of vessels that do not carry blood    *lymph(atic) vessels*
11. Abnormally slow heartbeat    *bradycardia*
12. External secretion    *exocrine*
13. Inflammation of the gallbladder    *cholecystitis*
14. Abnormal stoppage of menstruation    *amenorrhea*
15. A condition involving the white blood cells    *leukemia*
16. Science of the stomach and intestines    *gastroenterology*
17. Inflammation of a nerve    *neuritis*
18. Glands on top of the kidneys    *adrenal*
19. Inflamed condition of the brain    *encephalitis*
20. A minute arterial branch    *arteriole*
21. Situated upon a rib    *epicostal*

22. The terminal portion of the small intestine  *ileum*
23. Stem that refers to the blood vessels  *vascular*
24. Excision of a joint  *arthrectomy*
25. Without pain  *anesthesia (or analgesia)*

Definitions of the following terms and word elements are:

26. electrocardiogram  *written record of changes in the electrical potential of the heart*
27. epinephrine  *hormone secreted by the adrenal glands*
28. suffix  *added at the end of a word to further its meaning*
29. albuminuria  *presence of albumin in the urine*
30. endoparasite  *any parasite living within the body of another*
31. cystitis  *inflammation of the urinary bladder*
32. ab-  *prefix meaning off, away from*
33. a.c.  *before meals*
34. arthrocele  *a swollen joint*
35. epi-  *prefix meaning on, upon, about, beside*
36. dermatitis  *inflammation of the skin*
37. ilium  *a bone of the pelvic girdle (hip bone)*
38. cholelithiasis  *presence of gallstones*
39. asepsis  *sterile, clean*
40. ana-  *prefix meaning excessive or upward*
41. -oma  *suffix denoting a tumor or swelling*
42. anaerobe  *microorganism that grows without free oxygen*
43. enterocentesis  *surgical puncture of the intestines*
44. cardiovascular  *system of heart, arteries, veins, and capillaries*
45. aden-  *stem meaning glands*
46. abortion  *miscarriage, not a normal birth*
47. -em(ia)  *blood*
48. enteradenitis  *inflammation of the intestinal glands*
49. alb-  *white*
50. arthritis  *inflammation of the joints*

# Additional Exercise 2

(Answers to page 236)

The definitions are:

1. peripheral  *at or toward the surface of the body*
2. supine  *body lying on its back surface*

3. hyperglycemia   *an excess of blood sugar*
4. enterocentesis   *a surgical puncture into the intestines*
5. septicemia   *blood poisoning*
6. ventral   *at or near the front surface of the body*
7. prone   *lying face down and flat*
8. cholecystitis   *inflammation of the gallbladder*
9. arteriole   *a minute arterial branch*
10. amenorrhea   *abnormal stoppage of menstruation*
11. adduction   *to move toward the midline*
12. inferior   *toward the tail; beneath or below*
13. exocrine   *an external secretion (secreted into a duct)*
14. ostectomy   *removal of a bone*
15. epidermis   *the outer layer of skin*
16. hyperalgesia   *excessive sensitivity to pain*
17. leukemia   *a disease condition involving the white blood cells*
18. lateral   *at or near the side surface of the body*
19. adrenal   *glands on top of (near) the kidneys*
20. pyemia   *blood poisoning (characterized by pus formation)*
21. epicostal   *on top of a rib*
22. ileum   *the end portion of the small intestines*
23. dorsal   *at or near the back surface of the body*
24. encephalitis   *inflammation of the brain*
25. sagittal   *imaginary plane dividing the body from front to back into right and left sections*

# Additional Exercise 3

(Answers to page 237)

The prefix (P), root word (R), suffix (S), and definitions are:

1. colo/stomy   *opening created into the colon*
   **(R)**   **(S)**
2. hyper/adip/osis   *excessive condition of fat*
   **(P)**   **(R)**   **(S)**
3. my/oma   *tumor composed of muscle tissue*
   **(R)**   **(S)**
4. ost/emia   *congestion of blood in a bone*
   **(R)**   **(S)**

5. endo/card/itis    *inflammation of the lining of the heart*
   **(P)    (R)   (S)**
6. arthr/ectomy    *removal of a joint or part of joint*
   **(R)     (S)**
7. arter/itis    *inflammation of an artery*
   **(R)   (S)**
8. dermat/itis    *inflammation of the skin*
   **(R)     (S)**
9. hypo/tension    *abnormally low blood pressure*
   **(P)    (R)**
10. intra/hepatic    *within the liver*
    **(P)     (R)**
11. retro/sternal    *located behind the sternum*
    **(P)     (R)**
12. pre/operative    *before an operation*
    **(P)     (R)**
13. neuro/plasty    *surgery to repair or restore nerve function*
    **(R)      (S)**
14. quadri/plegia    *paralysis of all four limbs*
    **(P)      (R)**
15. dys/pnea    *difficult, painful breathing*
    **(P)    (R)**

# Additional Exercise 4

(Answers to page 238)

Definitions of the terms are:

1. lateral    *side surface of the body*
2. enteritis    *inflammation of the intestines*
3. hypoglycemia    *abnormally low blood sugar*
4. intravenous    *within a vein*
5. nephrocystitis    *inflammation of the kidneys and bladder*
6. craniotomy    *any surgical operation on the head*
7. supine    *body lying on its back surface*
8. bradycardia    *abnormally slow heartbeat*
9. postmortem    *after death*
10. colostomy    *artificial opening created in the colon*

11. encephalitis   *inflammation of the brain*
12. endocarditis   *inflammation of the lining of the heart*
13. ventral   *front surface of the body*
14. arthritis   *inflammation of a joint*
15. hyperthermia   *abnormally high body temperature*
16. hepatopexy   *surgery to reattach the liver to the abdominal wall*
17. gastroscope   *an instrument used to look into the stomach*
18. hemiplegia   *paralysis of one-half of the body (one side)*
19. dyspnea   *difficult, painful breathing*
20. appendectomy   *surgery to remove the appendix*
21. phlebitis   *inflammation of a vein*
22. retropleural   *located behind the lungs (pleural cavity)*
23. hemostat   *an instrument used to stop the flow of blood*
24. neurology   *the science and study of the nervous system*
25. arteriosclerosis   *hardening of the arteries*

Definitions of the prefixes are:

26. a-, an-   *not, without*
27. exo-   *outside of*
28. epi-   *on, upon, about, beside*
29. retro-   *behind, back*
30. hyper-   *excessive, too much*
31. intra-   *within*
32. peri-   *around*
33. anti-   *against*
34. dys-   *difficult, painful*
35. hypo-   *low, too little*

Definitions of the suffixes are:

36. -itis   *inflammation, infection of*
37. -ectomy   *surgical removal*
38. -otomy   *surgical incision*
39. -emia   *blood*
40. -plasty   *surgical repair, to form or build up*

Definitions of the stems are:

41. chole-   *bile, gallbladder*
42. cardi-   *heart*
43. aden-   *gland*
44. hepat-   *liver*
45. arthr-   *joint*

Definitions of the abbreviations are:

46. b.i.d.   *twice a day*
47. q4h   *every four hours*
48. h.s.   *at bedtime, hour of sleep*
49. I & O   *intake and output*
50. ua   *urinalysis*

# Crossword Puzzle #5 Answers

(Answers to page 240)

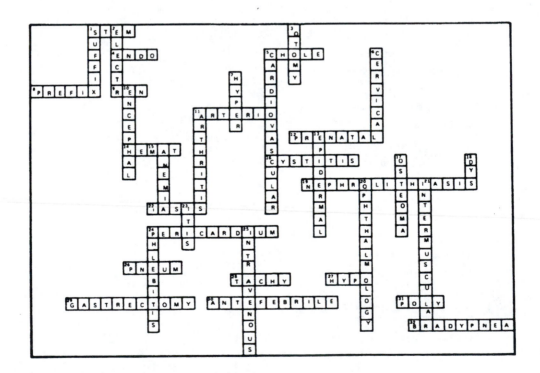

## Case History #1 Answers:

1. abdominal   *pertaining to the abdomen*
2. anorectal   *pertaining to the anus and rectum and the area between the two*
3. ED   *emergency department*
4. endoscopy   *an examination of an interior cavity of the body*
5. esophagitis   *an inflammation of the esophagus*
6. gastritis   *an inflammation of the stomach*
7. gastrointestinal   *pertaining to the stomach and intestines*
8. uropathy   *a disease change in the urinary tract*
9. mg   *milligrams*
10. q.d.   *every day*
11. t.i.d.   *three times a day*
12. p.r.n.   *as needed*
13. anemia   *lack of red blood cells*
14. chronic   *of long-lasting duration*
15. I.V. rehydration   *intravenous addition of fluids to the body*
16. q6h   *every 6 hours*
17. q24h   *every 24 hours*
18. I.M.   *intramuscularly*
19. sigmoidoscopy   *an examination of the sigmoid colon area of the intestines*
20. p.c.   *after meals*

## Discharge Summary Answers:

1. malignant   *becoming progressively worse*
2. hypertension   *elevated blood pressure*
3. WBC   *white blood cell count*
4. cardiomegaly   *enlarged heart, larger than normal*
5. pleural   *pertaining to the lungs*
6. renal   *pertaining to the kidneys*
7. hydronephrosis   *condition of a kidney swollen with too much urine (hydro = water, fluid)*
8. electrocardiogram   *a written record of the electrical activity of the heart*
9. ICU   *intensive care unit*
10. bilateral   *pertaining to two (or both) sides*
11. hemorrhage   *excessive flow of blood*
12. nephropathy   *disease in the kidneys*

# Posttest Solutions

(Answers to page 249)
1. **A.** before the stem
2. **C.** suffix
3. **A.** behind the breast bone
4. **B.** beneath the skin
5. **A.** the time period before the operation
6. **C.** after a meal
7. **B.** after death

8. n
9. g
10. j
11. i
12. l
13. k
14. q
15. u
16. c
17. w
18. o
19. f
20. e
21. x
22. m
23. h
24. h
25. p
26. b
27. e

28. **A.** without sensation
29. **C.** antidote
30. **B.** within a vein
31. **C.** outside a cell
32. white
33. red
34. away from
35. front

36. side surface
37. head
38. painful
39. night
40. prefix
41. much or frequent
42. few
43. hardening
44. swallow
45. removal
46. stem or root word
47. glands
48. skin
49. joint
50. heart
51. lungs
52. blood pressure
53. stomach
54. a large quantity of urine
55. **A.** a single form or shape
56. **B.** two points or cusps
57. **C.** three
58. **C.** four
59. **C.** many cells
60. **A.** paralysis of one lateral half of the body
61. **A.** around the heart
62. **C.** intercostal
63. **A.** alb-, **C.** leuk-
64. **B.** slow
65. **C.** tachycardia
66. **B.** low blood pressure
67. **A.** elevated blood pressure
68. an excess of
69. Cerebrology
70. prone
71. myoma
72. kidney
73. I.M.
74. -plasty
75. -cele

76. supine
77. caudal
78. colectomy
79. colostomy
80. protrusion, swelling
81. incision
82. enterectomy
83. gastritis
84. liver
85. kidney
86. bile, gallbladder
87. blood
88. fat or fatty
89. stones
90. kidneys
91. nerve
92. bone and joint
93. vein
94. suffix
95. tumor
96. infection
97. joint
98. vomiting
99. sharps
100. oncology

## Additional Resources

The following books are recommended for further study:

*Dorland's Illustrated Medical Dictionary,* 28th ed. W.B. Saunders, Philadelphia, PA, 1994.
    An extensive dictionary with numerous tables and excellent detailed illustrations.

*Learning Human Anatomy,* by Julia F. Guy, Appleton & Lange, Norwalk, CT, 1992.
    An easy-to-understand, well-illustrated, programmed text to further your understanding of the human body.

*Medical Terminology with Human Anatomy,* 3rd ed. by Jane Rice, Appleton & Lange, Norwalk, CT, 1995.
    Designed for a more advanced study of medical terminology including Spanish translation.

*Taber's Cyclopedic Medical Dictionary,* 17th ed. F.A. Davis Co., Philadelphia, PA, 1993.
    A smaller medical dictionary than Dorland's. Originally designed for nursing and allied health students.

    Some pharmaceutical companies have common medical terminology and abbreviation pamphlets available. Contact a sales representative in your area for copies.

    For a complete DRG listing, contact your regional office of the Health Care Finance Administration, listed in the phone book under Government Offices—United States Government, Department of Health and Human Services. The DRG listing is updated regularly in the Federal Register, usually in the fall.

# GLOSSARY

Alphabetical Listing of Word Elements Commonly Used
to Construct Medical Terms
Medical Specialties

# Alphabetical Listing of Word Elements Commonly Used to Construct Medical Terms

(Refer to the index for the page number where the word element is introduced. However, not all word elements listed are discussed in the text.)

| Element | Definition |
| --- | --- |
| **a-** | absent or deficient |
| **ab-** | away from |
| **abdomin-** | abdomen |
| **ac-** | to (see **ad-**) |
| **acr-** | extremity or peak |
| **ad-** | to (**d** changes to **c, f, g, p, s,** or **t** before stems beginning with these consonants) |
| **aden-** | gland |
| **adip-** | fat |
| **aer-** | air |
| **af-** | to (see **ad-**) |
| **ag-** | to (see **ad-**) |
| **-agra** | seizure of acute pain |
| **alb-** | white |
| **alg- (e) (o)** | relating to pain |
| **-algia** | painful condition |
| **all-** | other, different |
| **ambi-** | both |
| **amph- (i)** | doubly, both (the **i** is dropped before words beginning with a vowel) |
| **a-; an-** | without, not |
| **ana-** | upward, backward, excessive, or again (final **a** is dropped before words beginning with a vowel) |
| **andr- (o)** | relating to man |
| **angi- (o)** | relating to a blood vessel |

| | |
|---|---|
| **ant- (i)** | against |
| **ante-** | before (in time or place) |
| **ap-** | to (see **ad-**) |
| **arter- (i)** | artery |
| **arthr- (o)** | joint |
| **as-** | to (see **ad-**) |
| **at-** | to (see **ad-**) |
| **aur-** | ear |
| **auto-** | self |
| **aux-** | increase |
| **ax- (on)** | axis |
| **bi-** | two |
| **bio-** | life |
| **brachi-** | arm |
| **brachy-** | short |
| **brady-** | slow |
| **bronch-** | larger air passages within lungs |
| **calc- (l)** | stone |
| **carcin-** | cancer |
| **cardi-(o)** | heart |
| **caud-; caudal** | tail, away from the head, inferior |
| **cavity** | hollow space |
| **-cele** | tumor, hernia, swelling |
| **cente-** | puncture |
| **cephal-** | head |
| **cept-** | take, receive |
| **cerebr-** | cerebrum |
| **cervic-** | neck |
| **cheil-(o)** | lip |
| **chol-** | bile |
| **chondr-** | cartilage |

| | |
|---|---|
| **chro-** | color |
| **circum-** | around |
| **colo-** | colon |
| **co- (n, m, l, r)** | with, together |
| **contra-** | against, counter |
| **corp- (or)** | body |
| **cortic-** | bark, rind, outer layer |
| **cost-** | rib |
| **crani- (o)** | skull |
| **cranial** | pertaining to the head or skull |
| **cut-** | skin |
| **cyan-** | blue |
| **cyst- (o)** | sac, cyst, bladder |
| **cyt- (o)** | cell |
| **de-** | down, from |
| **dendr-** | tree |
| **dent-** | tooth |
| **derm- (a, at, o)** | skin |
| **-desis** | a binding |
| **di-** | two |
| **digit-** | finger, toe |
| **dipl- (o)** | double |
| **dis-** | apart, away from |
| **dors- (i); dorsal** | back |
| **duct-** | lead, conduct |
| **dur-** | hard |
| **dys-** | bad, improper |
| **e-** | out, from |
| **ect- (o)** | outside, without |
| **-ectomy** | excision of organ, or part |

| | |
|---|---|
| **electro-** | electricity |
| **-em-** | blood |
| **en-** | in, on (**n** changes to **m** before **b, p,** or **ph**) |
| **end-(o)** | inside |
| **enter-(o)** | intestine |
| **epi-** | upon, after, in addition (**i** is dropped before words beginning with a vowel) |
| **erythr-** | red |
| **ersthe-** | perceive, feel |
| **estr-(o)** | periodic changes in female reproductive organs |
| **ex-, (o)** | out of |
| **external** | outer part of a structure |
| **extra-** | outside of, beyond, in addition |
| **faci-(o)** | face |
| **fasci-** | band |
| **febr-** | fever |
| **fibr-** | fiber |
| **fil-** | thread |
| **flex-** | bent |
| **flux-; flu-** | flow |
| **for-** | opening |
| **-form** | shape |
| **fract-** | break |
| **front-** | forehead, front |
| **gangll-** | swelling, plexus |
| **gastr- (o)** | stomach |
| **gen-** | become, be produced, originate |
| **gest-** | bear, carry |
| **gloss-** | tongue |
| **-gram** | a writing, or record |
| **gran-** | grain, particle |

| | |
|---|---|
| **-graph** | draw, scratch, write, record |
| **grav-** | pregnant |
| **gyn (ec)-** | woman, female |
| **hem (at)-** | blood |
| **hemi-** | half |
| **hepat-** | liver |
| **hetero-** | other |
| **hist- (o), (io)** | tissue |
| **hom-** | common, same |
| **hydr- (o)** | water |
| **hyper-** | above, beyond, extreme |
| **hypo-** | under, below |
| **hyster-** | womb |
| **-ia** | state or condition |
| **idi-** | peculiar, separate, distinct |
| **ile-** | pertaining to the portion of the intestines known as the ileum |
| **ili-** | pertaining to the flaring part of the hip bone known as the ilium |
| **in-** | in, within, into, not, or negative |
| **inferior** | beneath, below |
| **infra-** | beneath |
| **inter-** | among, between |
| **internal** | inside of a structure |
| **intra-** | inside |
| **-ion** | process |
| **-itis** | denoting inflammation |
| **labi-** | lip |
| **lapar-** | flank or loin |
| **laryngo-** | windpipe |
| **later-; lateral** | side |
| **leuc-; (leuk-)** | white |

| | |
|---|---|
| **lingu-** | tongue |
| **lip-** | fat |
| **lith-** | stone |
| **-logy** | science of |
| **lute-** | yellow |
| **ly-** | loose, dissolve |
| **macr-** | large, long |
| **mal-** | bad, abnormal |
| **mast- (o)** | breast |
| **medi-; medial** | middle (midline) |
| **mega-** | great, large |
| **melan-** | black |
| **men-** | month |
| **mes-** | middle |
| **micr- (o)** | small |
| **mon- (o)** | one, single |
| **morph- (o)** | form, shape |
| **multi-** | many, much |
| **my- (o)** | muscle |
| **-myc (et) (es)** | fungus |
| **narc-** | numbness, stupor |
| **nas-** | nose |
| **ne- (o)** | new, young |
| **necr- (o)** | corpse, dead |
| **nephr- (o)** | kidney |
| **neur- (o)** | nerve |
| **nutri-** | nourish |
| **ob-** | against, toward, in front of (**b** changes to **c** before words beginning with **c**) |
| **oc-** | against (see **ob-**) |
| **ocul-** | eye |

| | |
|---|---|
| **odont- (o)** | tooth |
| **-oid** | resembling |
| **-oma** | tumor |
| **oo-** | egg |
| **ophthalm- (o)** | eye |
| **or-** | mouth |
| **orb-** | circle |
| **orchi-** | testicles |
| **orth-** | straight, right, normal |
| **oss-, os-, ost (e)-** | bone |
| **ot- (o)** | ear |
| **par-** | give birth to, bear |
| **para-** | beside, beyond (final **a** dropped before words beginning with a vowel) |
| **parietal** | wall of a structure |
| **path-** | that which undergoes sickness |
| **pec-; pex-** | fix, make fast |
| **pen-** | need, lack |
| **pept- (o)** | digestion |
| **per-** | through |
| **peri-** | around |
| **peripheral** | toward the surface of the body |
| **phag-** | eat |
| **pharyng-** | throat |
| **phleb- (o)** | vein |
| **phob-** | fear, dread |
| **phot- (o)** | light |
| **phren- (o)** | mind or diaphragm |
| **plas-** | mold, shape |
| **pne-** | breathing |
| **pneum (at)-** | lung/breath, air |

| | |
|---|---|
| **pneumo (n)-** | lung |
| **pod-** | foot |
| **poly-** | much, many |
| **post-** | after, behind in time or place |
| **pre-** | before in time or place |
| **pro-** | before in time or place |
| **proct-** | anus |
| **prone** | lying face down and flat |
| **proximal** | nearest the point of attachment |
| **pseud (o)** | false |
| **psych (o)** | mind, soul |
| **pto-** | fall, drop |
| **pulmo (n)** | lung |
| **py- (o)** | pus |
| **pyel- (o)** | trough, basin, pelvis |
| **quad(r)-** | four |
| **re-** | back, again |
| **ren (o)-** | kidney |
| **retro-** | backwards |
| **rhin (o)-** | nose |
| **-rrhage** | excessive flow |
| **-rhaphy** | suture |
| **-rrhea** | flow, or discharge |
| **-rrhexis** | rupture |
| **sanguin-** | blood |
| **sarc-** | flesh |
| **scler- (o)** | hard |
| **scop-** | look at or observe |
| **-sect** | cut |
| **sept-** | fence, wall off |
| **ser-** | watery substance |

| | |
|---|---|
| **-sis** | state or condition |
| **spas-** | draw, pull |
| **spin (o)-** | spine |
| **spondylo-** | denoting relationship to the spine |
| **-stalsis** | contraction |
| **sten- (o)** | narrow, compressed |
| **stom- (at) (ato) (o)** | mouth, orifice |
| **sub-** | under, below |
| **super-; superior** | above, addition, implying excess |
| **supra-** | above, upper, over |
| **supine** | lying on back surface |
| **syn-** | with, together |
| **tac** | order, arrange |
| **tachy-** | swift, rapid |
| **tens-** | stretch |
| **tetra-** | four |
| **therm (o)** | heat |
| **thorac- (o)** | chest |
| **thromb- (o)** | lump, clot |
| **tom- (y)** | cut |
| **tox-** | poison |
| **tract-** | draw, drag |
| **tri-** | three |
| **uni-** | one |
| **ur (o)-** | urine, urinary organs or tract |
| **vas-** | vessel |
| **ventral** | front |
| **visceral** | large interior organs; esp., the abdomen |
| **vit-** | life |
| **zyg (o)-** | union, join |

# Medical Specialties

A medical specialty is a branch of knowledge concerning a certain part of the body, its diseases, conditions, and treatments. A medical specialist is a doctor whose practice is devoted to a single branch of medical knowledge. Following are definitions of some of the more common medical specialties, given with the standard title of the physician practicing in those specialties.

**ALLERGY, ALLERGIST:** A subspecialty of internal medicine dealing with diagnosis and treatment of body reactions resulting from unusual sensitivity to foods, pollens, dusts, medicines, or other substances

**ANESTHESIOLOGY, ANESTHESIOLOGIST:** Administration of various forms of anesthesia in operations or diagnosis to cause loss of feeling, especially loss of the sensation of pain

**CARDIOVASCULAR DISEASES, CARDIOLOGY, CARDIOLOGIST:** A subspecialty of internal medicine involving the diagnosis and treatment of diseases of the heart and blood vessels

**DERMATOLOGY, DERMATOLOGIST:** Diagnosis and treatment of diseases of the skin

**GENERAL PRACTICE, GENERAL PRACTITIONER:** The diagnosis and treatment of disease by both medical and surgical methods, without limitation to organ systems or body regions, and without restriction as to the age of patients

**GENERAL SURGERY, SURGEON:** The diagnosis and treatment of disease by surgical means, without limitation to special organ systems or body regions

**GYNECOLOGY, GYNECOLOGIST:** Diagnosis and treatment of diseases of the female reproductive organs

**INTERNAL MEDICINE, INTERNIST:** The diagnosis and nonsurgical treatment of illnesses of adults

**NEUROLOGY, NEUROLOGIST:** Diagnosis and treatment of diseases of the brain, spinal cord, and nerves

**NEUROLOGICAL SURGERY, NEUROSURGEON:** Diagnosis and surgical treatment of brain, spinal cord, and nerve disorders

**OBSTETRICS, OBSTETRICIAN:** The care of women during pregnancy, childbirth, and the interval immediately following

**ONCOLOGY, ONCOLOGIST:** Diagnosis and treatment of tumors; a cancer specialist

**OPHTHALMOLOGY, OPHTHALMOLOGIST:** Diagnosis and treatment of diseases of the eye, including prescribing glasses

**OSTEOPATHY, OSTEOPATH:** Study and emphasis is in the theory that the body itself produces forces capable of fighting disease. Treatment is based on the musculoskeletal system and its alignment and may also include surgical and medicinal methods of diagnosis and therapy

**OTOLARYNGOLOGY, OTOLARYNGOLOGIST:** Diagnosis and treatment of diseases of the ear, nose, and throat

**PATHOLOGY, PATHOLOGIST:** Study and interpretation of changes in organs, tissues, and cells as well as alterations in body chemistry. These laboratory studies aid in diagnosing disease and determining treatment

**PEDIATRICS, PEDIATRICIAN:** Prevention, diagnosis, and treatment of children's diseases

**PLASTIC SURGERY, PLASTIC SURGEON:** Corrective or reparative surgery to restore deformed or mutilated parts of the body

**PSYCHIATRY, PSYCHIATRIST:** Diagnosis and treatment of mental disorders

**RADIOLOGY, RADIOLOGIST:** Use of radiant energy including x-rays, radium, cobalt 60, etc. in the diagnosis of disease

**THERAPEUTIC RADIOLOGY, RADIOLOGIST:** The use of radiant energy, including x-rays, radium, and other radioactive substances in the treatment of diseases

**THORACIC SURGERY, THORACIC SURGEON:** Operative treatment of the lungs, heart, and the large blood vessels within the chest cavity

**UROLOGY, UROLOGIST:** Diagnosis and treatment of diseases or disorders of the kidneys, bladder, ureters, urethra, and the male reproductive organs

# Index